Ann Burack-Weiss
Frances Coyle Brennan

Gerontological Supervision
A Social Work Perspective in Case Management and Direct Care

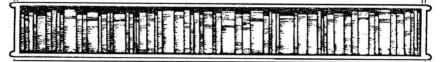

NOTES FOR PROFESSIONAL LIBRARIANS AND LIBRARY USERS

This is an original book title published by The Haworth Press, Taylor & Francis Group. Unless otherwise noted in specific chapters with attribution, materials in this book have not been previously published elsewhere in any format or language.

CONSERVATION AND PRESERVATION NOTES

All books published by The Haworth Press and its imprints are printed on certified pH neutral, acid-free book grade paper. This paper meets the minimum requirements of American National Standard for Information Sciences-Permanence of Paper for Printed Material, ANSI Z39.48-1984.

DIGITAL OBJECT IDENTIFIER (DOI) LINKING

The Haworth Press is participating in reference linking for elements of our original books. (For more information on reference linking initiatives, please consult the CrossRef Web site at www.crossref.org.) When citing an element of this book such as a chapter, include the element's Digital Object Identifier (DOI) as the last item of the reference. A Digital Object Identifier is a persistent, authoritative, and unique identifier that a publisher assigns to each element of a book. Because of its persistence, DOIs will enable The Haworth Press and other publishers to link to the element referenced, and the link will not break over time. This will be a great resource in scholarly research.

Gerontological Supervision

A Social Work Perspective in Case Management and Direct Care

Second Edition

Gerontological Supervision
A Social Work Perspective in Case Management and Direct Care

Second Edition

Ann Burack-Weiss
Frances Coyle Brennan

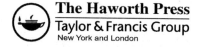
The Haworth Press
Taylor & Francis Group
New York and London

For more information on this book or to order, visit
http://www.haworthpress.com/store/product.asp?sku=5153

or call 1-800-HAWORTH (800-429-6784) in the United States and Canada
or (607) 722-5857 outside the United States and Canada
or contact orders@HaworthPress.com

Published by

The Haworth Press, Taylor & Francis Group, 270 Madison Avenue, New York, NY 10016.

PUBLISHER'S NOTE
The development, preparation, and publication of this work has been undertaken with great care. However, the Publisher, employees, editors, and agents of The Haworth Press are not responsible for any errors contained herein or for consequences that may ensue from use of materials or information contained in this work. The Haworth Press is committed to the dissemination of ideas and information according to the highest standards of intellectual freedom and the free exchange of ideas. Statements made and opinions expressed in this publication do not necessarily reflect the views of the Publisher, Directors, management, or staff of The Haworth Press, Inc., or an endorsement by them.

Identities and circumstances of individuals discussed in this book have been changed to protect confidentiality.

Second edition of *Gerontological Social Work Supervision* (The Haworth Press, 1991).

Cover design by Jennifer M. Gaska.

Library of Congress Cataloging-in-Publication Data

Burack-Weiss, Ann.
    Gerontological supervision : a social work perspective in case management and direct care / Ann Burack-Weiss, Frances Coyle Brennan.—2nd ed.
        p. cm.
    Rev. ed. of: Gerontological social work supervision / Ann Burack-Weiss, Frances Coyle Brennan.
    Includes bibliographical references.
    ISBN: 978-0-7890-2422-0 (hard : alk. paper)
    ISBN: 978-0-7890-2423-7 (soft : alk. paper)
    1. Social work with older people—United States. 2. Social workers—Supervision of—United States. I. Brennan, Frances Coyle. II. Burack-Weiss, Ann. Gerontological social work supervision. III. Title.

HV1465.B87 2007
362.6068'3—dc22

                                                                          2007033724

CONTENTS

ABOUT THE AUTHORS

Ann Burack-Weiss, DSW, LCSW, is an adjunct associate professor at the Columbia University School of Social Work. She is also a founding partner and co-director of SBW Partners, a firm that offers consultation, supervision, and training in the field of aging. She is the author of *The Caregiver's Tale: Loss and Renewal in Memoirs of Family Life,* co-author of *Social Work Practice with the Frail Elderly and Their Families,* and author of numerous chapters and journal articles. Her three decades of gerontological experience include practice, supervisory, and administrative positions.

Frances Coyle Brennan, LCSW, is the Director of Social Services at the Mary Manning Walsh Home in New York City. She was formerly an adjunct lecturer at Columbia University School of Social Work and is currently associated with Fordham University. She has over three decades of experience with the elderly in community and institutional settings, including supervisory and administrative positions at the Jewish Home and Hospital, and has written and presented extensively on issues in aging.

Ann Burack-Weiss and Frances Coyle Brennan are co-authors of *First Encounters Between Elders and Agencies: A Practice Guide* as well as the first edition of *Gerontological Social Work Supervision.*

Acknowledgments

Completion of a book is a time of remembrance and gratitude. Our first acknowledgment is to the countless social workers, social work interns, nurses, and gerontological supervisors in the New York City area with whom we have worked over the past three decades. Some were beginners. Others were experienced professionals. Some supervised one or two workers. Others administered large social service agencies or departments in health care settings. We worked together to integrate generic principles of practice and supervision to the field of gerontology. This book is a result of all that we have learned from them.

We are particularly grateful to the advisory group who offered us so much practice wisdom and support in preparation of this second edition. This outstanding group included Susannah Chandler, Barbara Rinehart, Valerie Ward, Sue Matorin, Chris Oates, Pat Blau, Laura Radensky, Tazuko Shibusawa, Renee Solomon, Lucy Rosengarten, and Lois Orlin. Our special thanks goes to Deirdre Downes for her careful reading and valuable suggestions to the manuscript.

We also thank our husbands, Roy L. Weiss and Tom Brennan, who helped turn our collaboration into many enjoyable times together. Our families, Donna Nelson, Danielle and Jennie Rose Nelson, Kenneth Weiss, Caroline and Tom Brennan, are an ongoing source of support and joy.

Gerontological Supervision
© 2008 by The Haworth Press, Taylor & Francis Group. All rights reserved.
doi:10.1300/5153_a

Part I:
An Overview

Chapter 1

Introduction

WHY A BOOK ON GERONTOLOGICAL SUPERVISION?

In 1991, we introduced the first edition of this book with a question: "Why a book on gerontological social work supervision?" We went on to explain the reasons that prompted us to write a book for master's level social work supervisors who worked with master's level social workers and graduate social work students in a range of settings that served the aged.

> For over a decade we have supervised, consulted with, and trained social workers in practice with the aging. During that time, we looked in vain for the literature that would offer us guidance. Finding none, we extrapolated from generic texts on supervision, literature on aging, and unpublished practice and supervisory wisdom of colleagues in the field.

Gerontological Supervision
© 2008 by The Haworth Press, Taylor & Francis Group. All rights reserved.
doi:10.1300/5153_01

Sometimes it all came together. Sometimes it did not. When it did, we could effectively prepare a young student, whose only previous exposure to aging was a globe-trotting grandmother, to enter a nursing home unit of Alzheimer's patients. When it did not, we were unable to help a middle-aged senior worker recognize that her identification with an adult daughter was distorting her assessment of an elderly couple's care needs.

In time, we were scoring more hits than misses. Clearly, there was something different about supervising practice with the aging, but exactly what? Was it merely that generic texts on supervision lacked case examples of gerontological practice, or something more?

We began writing this book without answers to that question. We reasoned that even if case examples of older people were sufficient to flesh out time honored supervisory principles, that in itself would provide justification for a new book. The rise in the elderly population and the increase in services to meet their needs are bringing thousands of new workers into agencies serving the aged each year. Social work supervisors with experience in other fields of practice are being called upon to administer and train staff in programs for older persons. Master's level social workers in aging are moving into supervisory positions within a year or two of graduation. Often, they have not conceptualized practice for themselves, much less thought about how to convey it to others.

So we began to write and, in the process, to discover something more. What makes supervising gerontological practice different is that the clients served not only could be, but will be, us. While other populations can arouse the compassion and even the identification of social workers, it is not the same. The social and health problems faced by other populations are disturbances in the natural course of events, anomalies of the human condition. Aging is the natural course of human events, the human condition. Social work students and workers may never know a schizophrenic, a substance abuser, or a developmentally delayed child outside of their professional work. But they will one day, if not today, be personally confronted with the issues that face their clients, both within their own families and for themselves. Supervision assumes an added dimension—that of helping workers— use their deepest human connection with aged clients and their families to the best professional end. (Burack-Weiss and Brennan, 1991, pp. 1-2)

CHANGES IN THE AGING FIELD OF PRACTICE

Fifteen years later, much of our thinking remains the same but the aging field of practice has changed. We now recognize that many of the growing population of people over sixty-five functions as independently as they did in midlife and are indistinguishable from other adult clients. Generic principles of practice and supervision require no alteration in meeting their needs.

At the same time, unprecedented numbers of older people with physical, cognitive, sensory, and emotional problems are flooding community services and long-term care settings—many of them being served by programs that did not exist when we wrote the first book. Two distinct roles have emerged in the provision of these services: the "case manager" and "the direct care worker." Often they work together or as part of a larger team that may include physicians, nurses, rehabilitation therapists, and other medical personnel.

The case manager is responsible for the overall progress and outcome of each case assigned to her. Her tasks usually include: engagement of client, assessment of client strengths and needs, contracting about the work to be done, developing a case plan, coordinating referrals within one's own agency and with outside agencies, counseling client and family, monitoring that all is going smoothly, reassessing and adjusting the plan as necessary, evaluating its effectiveness, and deciding if and when transfer or termination is necessary. The person who fills this role may be a bachelor or master's level social worker or a registered nurse. Occasionally this individual will have a college degree but no professional training.

The direct care worker is responsible for hands-on care to the older person. In a long-term care setting, she most likely will be called a "nursing assistant." In the community, she may be known as a "home health aide" or "home attendant." Unlike the case manager whose contact with the client rarely exceeds one hour a week (and most often is less) the direct care worker will spend hours each day helping the older person with such intimate activities as bathing, dressing, feeding, and toileting. In the community, her tasks may expand to cleaning, shopping, laundry, cooking, and escort services. The relevant education of the person who fills this role is typically restricted to agency-based training. Because her contact with the client is so frequent and close, the direct care worker often becomes the personification of help to the older person.

Most community and long-term care programs that offer services to ill or disabled older people designate a professionally credentialed staff member (usually an MSW or RN but occasionally an individual with a degree in gerontology, public health, public administration, or education) to the position of supervisor—charged with ensuring that case managers and direct care workers carry out the agency mandate while meeting reimbursement and certification requirements.

Today, it is not unusual for supervisors to find themselves responsible for the work of staff members with different professional training and orientations than their own. A nurse may supervise a social worker. A social worker may supervise a nurse. Professionals who supervise direct care workers may have limited experience with the difficult tasks and emotional demands of the job.

Added to these difficulties is the current climate of gerontological services that places enormous pressures on agencies to be cost-effective—resulting in larger caseloads, less time to each case, and less supervisory time for each worker. Management focus is often on statistics, such as how many older people receive how many hours of service, by how many service providers. Sufficient thought is rarely given to the ways in which these services are delivered—the quality of care that older people receive and how we can foster humane, appropriate care delivery through implementing educational, supportive, and administrative supervision strategies to frontline workers.

As the greatest need for gerontological supervisory skill is currently in settings serving ill and disabled older people, and the fact that such supervision is cross-disciplinary, multilevel, and subject to greater outside pressures than ever before, we have decided to widen the reach of the second edition to nonsocial workers while maintaining what we call "a social work perspective." Four interrelated concepts frame the perspective and underlie all the chapters that follow: parallel process, the power of relationship, a holistic approach, and a dual emphasis on the person and the environment. These concepts are amplified in Chapter 2.

ABOUT THE BOOK

This book reflects the experience that each of us has amassed in over three decades of gerontological practice. During this time, we have provided direct services to older people and their families as well as training, supervision, and consultation to all levels of staff in a range of community and institutional care settings in the New York City area. As this area reflects enormous diversity, we believe that our ideas are applicable to a range of geographical and practice settings.

Gerontological Supervision: A Social Work Perspective in Case Management and Direct Care is filled with direct and composite examples from our own experience and that of colleagues, interns, and supervisees. In no way a compendium of supervisory approaches, research findings, or academic theory, it fits more aptly into a category that was once called "practice wisdom"—a passing on of what we have learned to those who are setting out on the road we have traveled.

We owe a great debt to past and present theoreticians. From the works of Bertha Reynolds and Charlotte Towle, we incorporate the philosophical and psychodynamic roots of supervision. These early works on supervision remind us that the supervisee is a person with unique characteristics and life experiences. They alert us to the need for individualization, respect for learning style, and awareness of the sequential stages of the learning process. Inductively based on these writers' own personal experiences, the supervisory principles embedded in these works have a timeless truth that outlasts the agency services on which they are based.

Current literature on supervision is more often empirically based and cognizant of the impact of the agency's organizational structure on practice. Here, we have drawn most frequently on the works of Alfred Kadushin, Carlton E. Munson, and Lawrence Shulman. They have helped us to identify what is indeed generic to all good supervisory practice and what must be modified to meet the needs of specific agencies and populations. (We are particularly appreciative of the work of Lawrence Shulman who has creatively adapted the seminal theories of William Schwartz to the interactional process of supervision.)

The case examples that appear in these pages might make it appear that every problem has a satisfactory solution and that it is the supervisor's fault if things do not turn out well. Nothing could be further from the truth. Sometimes, despite one's best efforts, the older person cannot be helped or the worker must be terminated. As there are so many intervening variables over which they have no control, supervisors may not be able to influence the outcome of a situation. What they can influence is the process. We hope that the processes inherent in our discussion and examples will lead readers to creative applications of their own.

Those who are familiar with the first edition will note that much of the content remains the same. However, we have made significant changes by eliminating some old material, shuffling the rest, and adding new ideas and case examples. We have moved from a focus on programs serving all the elderly to those that serve ill or disabled older people. Moving from an exclusive focus on MSW students and staff to those with other professional training—or no professional training at all—we have adapted the text and the book title accordingly.

Part I (Chapters 1-4) provides an overview of the social work perspective on gerontological supervision as well as a discussion of the principles on which it is based. This section—applicable to supervising all levels of staff—presents the stages and styles of helping, learning, and teaching.

Part II (Chapters 5-7) addresses practice issues involved in the supervision of social workers and case managers. This section discusses ways to help workers acquire the necessary skills to intervene effectively with elders, their families, and other health and social service providers.

Part III (Chapters 8-10) addresses administrative issues involved in the supervision of social workers and case managers. It includes a discussion of organizational opportunities and constraints, training, group supervision, evaluation, and the conduct of "difficult conversations."

Part IV (Chapters 11-13) is devoted to all aspects of the supervision of interns. Although it is based on a social work model of field education, we believe it can be adapted to students in other helping professions.

Part V (Chapters 14-17) is an addition to the first edition. It discusses the commonalities and differences involved in supervising direct care workers in home care and long-term care settings as well as a discussion of training, group supervision, and evaluation for this essential group of service providers.

Chapter 2

The Social Work Perspective

The social work perspective on gerontological supervision is based on four interrelated concepts: parallel process, the power of relationship, a holistic approach, and a dual emphasis on person and environment. These concepts rest on a set of values that are shared with other health care providers: seeking strengths, promoting optimum functioning, promoting the least restrictive environment, promoting ethical conduct, treatment with dignity and respect, developing cultural competence, and setting appropriate goals.

PARALLEL PROCESS

The dictionary defines "process" as "a series of actions over time." Parallel process refers to the fact that the supervisor's ongoing interactions with the worker are based on the same values and use many of the same skills, as the practitioner's work with clients—and may even serve as a model for that work.

Parallel process speaks of the capacities of clients and workers to change and to learn if given time and space to do so. A frail older person who lives in a cluttered unsafe environment is unlikely to change lifelong habits on the basis of a onetime discussion. A worker who is combative with others on her team will rarely change her approach on the basis of one supervisory conference. However, that is no reason to give up on a client or on a worker. Exploration of their thoughts and feelings, recognition of their doubts, appreciation of their strengths, sensitive timing of suggestions, and support as they accept new ways of being usually pays off—even if it may take longer than outsiders think it should.

Gerontological Supervision
© 2008 by The Haworth Press, Taylor & Francis Group. All rights reserved.
doi:10.1300/5153_02

THE POWER OF RELATIONSHIP

The relationship is the medium through which all help flows. Strong relationships—between supervisors and workers, workers and clients, and workers and families—are rarely devoid of conflict. Differences of opinion are bound to occur. The inherent authority of one individual who has power over another may sometimes breed resentment, if not rebellion. The worker balks at an assigned task. The client refuses to accept services that the agency feels is necessary to ensure her safety. The power of these relationships is in the human connection and trust that underlies the issue of the moment.

The supervisor can demonstrate how one can offer care and support while keeping a focus on case objectives and worker goals. This is done by getting "taboo" topics out in the open, nonjudgmentally discussing opposing views of a problem, living with the anxiety of unresolved situations and the pain of irrevocable losses, exercising authority in a respectful manner, accepting when she has made a mistake, apologizing, and moving on. In so doing, she will model a "professional use of self" that the worker will often unconsciously echo in her work with clients.

As we believe so strongly in the efficacy of parallel process and the power of relationship in achieving both practice and supervisory goals, we illustrate most portions of this text by showing how our ideas play themselves out in both situations.

A HOLISTIC APPROACH

A holistic approach—one that integrates understanding of the physical, psychological, social, and cultural situation of client or worker—is an essential component of the social work perspective on gerontological supervision. The illness or disability of the client and the job-related problem of the worker must be understood in the context of their life experiences. This is not to say that older clients necessarily need psychodynamic counseling or that a therapeutic model should prevail in supervision. (Appropriate boundaries must be set and upheld in both situations.) Rather, it is to recognize that understanding people means taking into account their beliefs and preferences, and the impact that factors such as age, gender, race/ethnicity, and sexuality have on their world view. Above all, a holistic approach means going beyond the cataloging of problem areas to recognizing and mobilizing strengths in the elder and the worker.

DUAL EMPHASIS ON PERSON AND ENVIRONMENT

Social work is unique among professions in its emphasis on improving the interaction between individuals and the environments in which they live. The elder is composed of systems (physical, psychological, social, and cultural) and his environment is constituted of systems (family, friends, neighbors, and helping organizations). As services to ill and disabled older people involve multiple environmental systems and forces, social work's dual emphasis on person and environment is particularly relevant to gerontological practice and supervision.

Case managers and social workers typically spend as much time in negotiating with service providers, participating in team conferences, and working with family members, neighbors, and friends as they do in face-to-face interactions with the older person. Direct care workers—especially in the community—are often charged with speaking up for their clients or interpreting their wishes to others. Helping elders achieve the highest level of functioning possible means that both case managers and direct care workers must work to empower individuals to act on their own behalf whenever they are able to do so as well as mediate and advocate when external support is needed.

The social work perspective is based on commonly held values about the goals and processes of practice with the elderly. All of the guiding principles presented in this chapter are elaborated further in the chapters that follow.

SEEKING STRENGTHS

In Practice

Agencies and funding sources ask the worker to identify the client's problems. Good practice requires the worker to identify and mobilize client strengths. Dormant capacities for pleasure and survival developed through a lifetime can be reactivated by a creative worker who

finds out how the older person coped in the past. A blind and paralyzed man on a skilled nursing unit may retain the interest and cognitive capacity to follow world news if a radio is brought to his bedside.
A frail, arthritic woman in the community can continue to demonstrate
love for her visiting family by making their favorite soup if the home
care attendant shops for and readies all the ingredients in advance.

Often a client's strength shows itself in difficult behavior. A nursing home resident who is constantly asking for special attention from
the nurses may be asserting his individuality in what he perceives as a
dehumanizing experience. The worker who can identify the strength
and redirect it appropriately has performed a valuable service to staff
as well as to client.

In Supervision

The supervisor can alert workers to client strengths by asking them
to focus on what is right, rather than what is wrong in any given situation. What does the older person have going for him? For one, it may
be an engaging personality that makes others volunteer to help her.
For another, it may be a lifelong habit of perseverance that pays off in
his ability to sustain a taxing program of physical therapy. Identifying
the ways in which the ill or disabled person survived the challenges of
the past and helping him to use these strengths to meet the current
challenge can be a gratifying experience for all levels of staff.

A worker might also have strengths that are not immediately apparent or show themselves in difficult behavior. An intern might have mu-
sical or artistic skills that can be used with nonverbal clients. A direct
care worker who balks at using the feeding methods a case manager
suggests may have developed a better approach from her previous work
experience. Asking workers about their previous life and work experiences that are relevant to the job at hand often yields useful results.

PROMOTING OPTIMUM FUNCTIONING

In Practice

The task with older people who have sustained physical or mental
losses is to help them achieve and maintain the highest level of functioning possible given their disability. This is done by assessing how

physical, psychological, social, and cultural factors interact in the older person's performance of life-sustaining and life-enhancing activities. It is not enough to focus solely on the person, environmental supports are also needed. An elder who cannot climb stairs will be disabled if her apartment is on the third floor of a walk-up building. An elder who can no longer drive will be disabled if there is no other transportation available to take him to appointments. Their functioning will improve dramatically if needed supports and services are provided.

In Supervision

Supervisors have a vital role in promoting maximum functioning in their workers and the clients they serve. Although "independence" is often cited as a goal, achieving "interdependence" is more relevant. Neither workers nor clients should feel that doing the best they can for themselves will result in withdrawal of support when the going gets tough. The good supervisor knows that the individual who performs at optimum level one day might have problems the next day. Observing when others need a hand and stepping in—even taking over—for a time is sometimes indicated. The case manager who has trouble presenting agency policy to an angry family member might benefit from having the supervisor at her side. The direct care worker who can handle an agitated Alzheimer's patient within her apartment might need a back-up person when they go to the hospital clinic where there is a long wait to be seen.

PROMOTING THE LEAST RESTRICTIVE ENVIRONMENT

In Practice

Although the concept of least restrictive environment is essentially a legal one it applies directly to ill or disabled older people. Society accepts the rights of individuals to live as they wish unless they pose a threat to themselves or to others. In such situations, individual freedom is abrogated only to the extent necessary to remove the threat.

The notion of least restrictive environment is closely related to the idea of parsimony in medical and social interventions. One intrudes as little as possible to achieve the desired end. Outpatient medical procedures are preferable to hospital admissions; home care is considered before nursing home placement.

The issues are rarely clear-cut. Ascertaining the presence and degree of risk is subjective. Older people who are mentally competent may willingly accept the risks of living alone that are unacceptable to their families and health care providers. Older people who are not mentally competent pose even greater dilemmas.

Suppose an older woman wishes to remain in her own apartment but has grown so confused that she has been seen outside on scorching summer days wrapped up in a winter coat. Is her behavior sufficient reason to declare incompetence and place her in a nursing home against her will? Court appointed conservators or family members with power of attorney may call on the case manager for direction. And she will turn to her supervisor.

In Supervision

When case managers are faced with decisions that have no right answer they need the supervisor's counsel and support in thinking out the consequences of each option. The supervisory role assumes special administrative importance because of the agency's potential liability if a client or an innocent bystander is injured.

Often a compromise can be worked out. In the case described, full-time home care may seem a desirable intervention but be rejected by the client who will only agree to a few hours of service a day. Knowing that the agency is committed to building up the support system and receiving frequent progress reports may preserve the client's rights as well as calm those calling for an immediate, drastic solution.

Workers sometimes protest that demands of the workplace restrict their ability to do their jobs as well as they could. (Paperwork takes time away from seeing clients, agency policy and procedures inhibit their creativity, and having their work frequently checked is an indication that they are not trusted.) Rather than reacting with defensiveness or anger, the supervisor might ask herself how much leeway for individual discretion is actually possible within the agency. While most job rules and regulations are nonnegotiable, there are always a few that can be applied differentially. Greater work autonomy may be granted to senior staff than to newcomers, or workers can be asked rather than told about what time schedule for meeting assigned tasks works best for them.

It might also be the case that staff are protesting what they see as a lack of recognition for "doing more with less" that has become the norm in many health-related settings. At a time when everyone—including supervisors—feels pressured and unappreciated, simple recognition that staff complaints are valid (even if not open to amelioration) and support through a difficult time is helpful.

PROMOTING ETHICAL CONDUCT

In Practice

Ethical considerations in work with the aged are not limited to end-of-life decisions or situations of overt worker malpractice. Violations are often subtle or so frequent that they become accepted without notice. Hurried staff in medical clinics often ask older people to sign "Informed Consent" forms that contain print too small to read or incomprehensible phrases they do not take time to explain.

The need for confidentiality is also frequently bypassed under the assumption that ill or disabled older people will not know or will not care that information about them is shared. Thus agencies may communicate over the phone about a case without first obtaining a signed release. Direct care workers may share privileged information they have learned about clients and families with people in the neighborhood or co-workers in a residential setting.

Ill and disabled older people must often trade a measure of privacy for the help they receive. Financial concerns, personal habits, and sexual practices that were once nobody else's business are suddenly open to view. Frail elders who have no concerned family or friends are apt to arouse feelings of compassion in their workers who want to step in and act as surrogate relatives. Boundaries between client and worker are liable to become blurred. Maintaining these boundaries without sacrificing the human connection that is a vital part of the helping process is a challenge for most workers in the field.

In Supervision

It is not always easy to differentiate an ethical problem from a practice problem. Practice problems can be resolved by helping a worker expand her knowledge base and develop new skills. Frequently, two opposing positions are presented as an "ethical dilemma." An example would be the client's right to know his terminal diagnosis versus the family's desire that he is spared the truth. Rather than entering into a philosophical discussion, the supervisor can explore how much the worker knows about the thoughts and fears of all involved, what communication she has fostered within the family, her understanding of ambivalence, and the fact that everyone's point of view is liable to change. Armed with new insights and skills, the worker may be able to return to the family and resolve the situation.

That said, there are true ethical dilemmas. A client may be happy to accept some agency services but reject others that have been deemed essential to his safety and health. He is exercising his right to self-determination. The agency of record may also exercise its right to discontinue all services rather than participate in a dangerous situation for which they could be held responsible. A skillful case manager might be able to help the client understand the consequences of his decision. A skillful supervisor might be able to advocate with the agency for a delay hoping that a better solution can be found. However, even when a satisfactory resolution to the dilemma is not achieved, the worker who feels that the supervisor is on her side will be more apt to trust her with other ethical and practice concerns.

Although informed consent, confidentiality, self-determination, and boundaries are fine topics for staff training or development sessions, these values are more often "caught" than "taught." The supervisor who consistently demonstrates these qualities with her workers has taken the first step in making them aware of their importance.

TREATMENT WITH DIGNITY AND RESPECT

In Practice

Treating ill or disabled older people with dignity and respect is more than the absence of restraints and first-rate physical care. It is honoring their personhood in small but significant ways.

This involves:

Knocking before entering a room or opening a closed door.

Addressing the elder by her last name unless asked to do otherwise. (This includes not using "young lady," "Momma," "Pops," or other made-up terms of mock affection.)

Allowing choices when choices are possible. (Rather than telling the client what time the case manager will be making a home visit, a choice between a few possible hours will send the message that her time and schedule is respected.)

Including the elder in every conversation that takes place around him. This applies when more than one direct care worker is involved in escorting, feeding, or bathing elders. It also applies to case managers holding family conferences. (Demented clients pick up much on a sensory level; soft touches and reassuring voices are important.)

Protecting the elder's privacy in intimate moments of care: such as toileting and bathing. (Extra sheets, towels, and screening are not cosmetic extras but essential signs of respect.)

Sitting down to speak with chair or bed-bound elders rather than standing above them. (Even if the contact is only for a minute or two, it will seem longer and the elder will feel valued.)

In Supervision

Dignity and respect for clients is demonstrated through recognizing and reversing common situations in which it is violated. Dignity and respect for workers is similarly shown.

It begins with recognition that the supervisory role carries power. Added to the power differential within the relationship itself is the larger society in which it is embedded. As much as supervisors and workers may reject or resist these strictures—privileging men over women, the well-off over the poor, Caucasians over other races (even the concept of race itself), midlife adults over the young or the old, heterosexuality over homosexuality, the better educated over the less educated, and native born Americans over immigrants—all the stereotypes and judgments that accompany these dimensions of difference are present in the room when client and worker or supervisor and worker meet. Direct care workers usually hold a one-down position along several of the dimensions by which people are judged in society and a sense of a devalued status often influences their interactions with the supervisor.

The supervisor who recognizes "the elephant in the room" and asks the worker how it might affect their interaction will usually be met with denial. However, the words have been said and heard, and the topic once opened, is more easily opened again.

DEVELOPING CULTURAL COMPETENCE

In Practice

The aging population represents greater ethnic and cultural diversity than any other in the United States today. Not only have older immigrants arrived from the four corners of the world bringing their beliefs, customs, and practices with them; but fully assimilated Americans often return to cultural roots and mother tongues as they grow older. Attitudes toward receiving help, institutionalization, illness, and family responsibilities (among others) vary considerably among nationalities. The cultural component is fundamental in every client assessment.

At a time when Hispanic, Asian, Caucasian, and African-American elders hail from a variety of countries, each with its own politics, cultural history, and customs (often its own language) no one can be expected to know it all. What is the worker to do? Glossing over differences in the belief that basic values and needs of all elders are essentially alike may seem the least prejudicial, most accepting approach. This method can deprive elders of their unique differences and strengths when they most need affirmation. However, emphasis on the cultural characteristics of various aging populations can easily deteriorate into caricatures and stereotypes that do an equal disservice.

The social work maxim to "begin where the client is" is particularly applicable to developing cultural competence. Admitting that one does not know about the elder's background and is interested in hearing about it is an important first step. As elders tell of how their parents lived their last years, the kind of care provided to them, and what they expected in turn, the worker gets a clearer picture of their belief systems.

Independence is widely regarded as a sign of adulthood and the newly dependent elderly are often struggling with a perceived, and often actual, drop in status. In many cultures, having to go outside the family (or even the cultural community) for help is a strategy of last resort and many elderly feel ashamed to have come to this point.

Other aspects of culture—such as food preferences and ritual practices—should also be explored. After asking about a client's culture and actively listening to the responses, the worker can turn to the literature (now widely available through journals and the Web) to fill in.

In Supervision

Workers need to see *themselves* as cultural beings—who bring to practice many unexamined cultural assumptions about how the world works and their own place in it. This is as true of the financially struggling African-American direct care worker assigned to an upper middle-class Caucasian client as it is when an Asian middle-class case manager is assigned to a poor Latina client. While these workers rarely have trouble perceiving biases and prejudices toward themselves, they might have greater difficulty accepting their own culturally rooted notions as affecting their assessments and interactions. Modeling the accepting, focused exploration of culture she expects of her workers, the supervisor can explore with her workers. What was their family's experience with its older relatives? How does their culture view proper behavior toward the elderly, family responsibility, and end-of-life experiences? Preceding this discussion with an explanation of its relevance to practice—and following it with a request that the worker take some time to reflect upon it—reinforces the message. Staff training and development on cultural competence, as well as readings, are a useful adjunct but cannot substitute for the worker's inward journey. As discussed at length in Part V—groups are a particularly useful forum for direct care workers to share their thoughts and feelings about differences and similarities between their culture and those of their clients.

SETTING APPROPRIATE GOALS

In Practice

One often hears of the importance of setting limited goals for ill or disabled elders—as if clients of other ages and statuses were not limited in some way by their personalities and environment. It is more useful to think of goals as being appropriate to the circumstances and wishes of the client. Workers usually try to maintain a current level of functioning or adaptation to a lower level of functioning more often than radical change or growth. Nevertheless, there are opportunities for clients to thrive and workers to be gratified with a job well done.

Good practice promotes life-sustaining and life-enhancing interventions. No one gets up in the morning only to dress, wash, or perform any of the other "activities of daily living" with which service providers are often preoccupied. While we must help clients perform these tasks they are a means to an end, not ends in themselves. Gerontological workers must seek and promote those individualized sources of satisfaction that give their clients reasons to survive.

In Supervision

As workers with the elderly acknowledge the importance of "activities of daily living" while looking beyond them to individual sources of satisfaction they can help their clients achieve, so, the supervisor can look beyond the fulfillment of job requirements to the individual supervisee.

The supervisor is in a unique position to identify worker strengths and help them set their own goals for professional or career development—apart from the goals that have been set for them in their current positions. For one it may be further education. For another, it may be consolidating the skills they already have or being promoted within the agency. Being attuned to the goals of individual workers and finding ways they can meet them within the jobs they currently occupy is a humane as well as an effective supervisory strategy.

Chapter 3

Stages of Helping, Learning, and Teaching

ABOUT DEPENDENCE

In Practice

We live in a society that values independence and autonomy. Adults are expected to handle their own finances, plan and carry out their own life activities, maintain their homes, and care for their own personal needs. Even when individuals choose to delegate some of these responsibilities, they maintain control. The situation changes when age-related losses render them dependent on others—especially when these others are not family members but strangers who are paid to care.

Familiar, comforting routines are upset. Privacy is intruded upon. The very act of leaning on another for decisions and help with intimate tasks is a constant reminder of how far they are now removed from their former lives—a realization that is reinforced when they must move from their own homes into an institutional setting.

There are some ill and disabled elders who recognize that they need help and are appreciative when it is offered; and there are others whose cognitive deficits obscure or mute the effect of dependence. However, older people who retain awareness of their situations suffer some diminishment of self-esteem when they need help accomplishing tasks they used to handle on their own.

No longer feeling in control over their own living situations (or even the performance of daily tasks) some elders lash out at those who try to help with the only power they feel is left to them—the power of refusal. The battlegrounds of this fight for independence may appear

Gerontological Supervision
doi:10.1300/5153_03

minor (the refusal to take a bath or to get dressed) but they represent some measure of control to the ill or disabled older person who feels powerless. Others may project their anger over being dependent on those who care for them. Perpetually unhappy with the help they receive—and physically or verbally abusing those who try to offer it—they alienate all who come near them. Still others withdraw into themselves—in sadness and passivity, or become overly clinging and more dependent than their situation would warrant.

In Supervision

Workers have their own issues related to dependence. Some are related to maintaining a compassionate yet professional demeanor with clients who depend on them for so much. Others arise from the supervisory relationship itself.

The worker often spends more time alone with the client—and gets to know him more intimately—than do many of his family members. The powerful human bond with a caring figure may, in the long run, be as influential as physical care or concrete services in helping ill and disabled elders find meaning and satisfaction in their lives. At the same time, there are dangers.

The worker who is seen, and sees herself, as "one of the family" may be unable to separate herself from the problems of a client to perform her role professionally. She will have less to offer other clients under her care, find the work situation intruding on her personal life, and is a likely candidate for burnout. What is more, her efforts to help may involve taking on more of the work than is necessary, unwittingly rendering the client more dependent than he needs to be. Just as problematic is the worker who protects herself from getting "too close" by emotionally distancing herself from the client—especially a client who hungers for personal warmth in the relationship.

As noted throughout this book, the supervisory relationship mirrors that of the client and worker. Workers sometimes appreciate, sometimes chafe against dependence on supervisory direction. Like their clients, they may know they need direction and nurturing while at the same time wishing that they did not.

The supervisor also struggles with when and how to step in. Is it better to offer less guidance, to let the worker make—and learn from her own mistakes? Or is it in the best interest of worker and client to anticipate difficulties and head them off? Individual assessment of the worker's place along the continuum of stages and styles of learning provides guidance.

RESPONSES TO DEPENDENCY AND LOSS

Common human responses accompany dependency and loss of control in ill and disabled older people. They are shock/disbelief, denial, bargaining, anger and sadness, and negotiating the balance between independence and dependence. We believe that responses to dependence and loss of control are also present, to some degree, in the workers who bear witness to them. Not everyone will experience every response in a predictable sequence; however, an understanding of what may arise can prepare the supervisor for what, on the surface, may seem inexplicable behavior on the part of clients or workers.

Shock and Disbelief

In Practice

Aging is a continuous process, and old age is an anticipated status. Nevertheless, the dawning of awareness is an individual and shocking occurrence often occasioned by a specific event: a medical diagnosis, the funeral of a contemporary, or the chance remark of a stranger. At first, these are fleeting moments soon dwarfed by other experiences, but as the moments accumulate the reality is ever present.

There is disbelief in the changing body so at odds with the inner self, shock at the often insidious lack of respect accorded to older people in our culture, and surprise at the paucity of help available in times of need.

The individual for whom the reality of old age has just set in needs time to come to terms with his feelings and options. What experiences can be harnessed to meet present-day demands? What new activities or interests can offer gratification? This sorting process does not usually take place on a conscious level. Most often, it can be inferred by observation of the elder's trial and error efforts at mastery.

In Supervision

Practitioners new to the field of aging also need time to get their bearings. Myths and certainties about aging are debunked one by one leaving uncertainty and ambiguity in their wake. A process of sorting out occurs as the new practitioner struggles to overcome erroneous beliefs and assimilate new learning. Stereotypes and generalizations about who old people are, what they need, and how to help them, are assaulted by the individual client who defies easy understanding.

The case manager or intern who anticipated friendly visits during which concrete services would be provided to appreciative older people will be surprised by the hostility and pathology that is as present in this population as any other. The direct care worker who anticipated that the aged she would be caring for would be like older members of her family or community may be challenged by lifestyles, attitudes, and beliefs so different from her own.

Case managers, interns, or direct care workers may handle their anxiety by seeking answers to hypothetical situations. Or they may become self-critical, questioning their own abilities to do what has to be done. Some will cling tightly to previous beliefs—asking for validation, supervisory opinion that they are "right" in their expectations.

The strategies that work with the elder in shock and disbelief are equally effective with practitioners. The aim is to shore up the ego; to put clients and workers in touch with their strengths and resources as well as experiences that can be called upon to meet a new challenge.

As supportive counseling is most effective with the older person going through a period of shock and disbelief, supportive supervision is the approach of choice for the new worker. The goal in both cases is noninterference with the individual's natural processes of adaptation and ultimately the mastery of new circumstances. The goal is to focus worker's attention on what they *can* do to help, even at this stage of inexperience; to respond to the worker's feelings of inadequacy by providing concrete information and support.

Denial

In Practice

Every practitioner has known the aged client who does not want to be with "those old people." In fact, congregate services in the community and moving to senior living situations are often spurned for that reason. Denial also appears in more subtle guises; noncompliance with a medical regime, refusal of necessary services, and habitual interactions with others that are no longer appropriate.

Denial can be functional in old age. Refusal to acknowledge a loss may actually contribute to successful adaptation in situations where nothing can or must be done. It is only when denial interferes with needed care that it must be challenged.

In Supervision

Practitioners may also exhibit denial. Troubled by the specifics of the case before them, they cling to general beliefs. The case manager who resolves that the aged are like everyone else will deny cohort, sensory, or cognitive differences to make the individual case fit into practice models she has learned at school or with other populations. The direct care worker who has fixed ideas about how activities of daily living should be accomplished may deny the difficulty aged clients have in complying with her schedule.

At the other extreme is the practitioner who resolves that the aged are a special case for whom a professional approach is irrelevant. The case manager, intern, or direct care worker may enter into an ambiguous social relationship with the client or act as a surrogate child, promoting confusion in the relationship.

Supporting the elder's and practitioner's positive coping attempts while explaining the reality is the first step. Both client and worker may first respond with anger or even greater denial. However, the mere statement of reality helps them begin to consider alternative ways of handling the situation.

The task of the supervisor at this stage is to help workers discover what general knowledge base is applicable and what must be altered in their work with the aged. While the denial of the older person is best addressed by a clear statement and reenforcement of reality supported by a caring worker, the denial of the worker is most profitably challenged by didactic teaching and assigned readings by a caring supervisor.

Bargaining

In Practice

The recognition of loss and all the painful feelings associated with it is usually gradual and intermittent. As loss enters the older person's consciousness, a period of bargaining may ensue. One older person will accept transportation and escort to medical appointments but not a home attendant. Another might be fine with a high intensity lamp to improve vision but not accept the outdoor cane that would identify her as blind.

Awareness of what is irrevocably lost is sinking in, and the older person is testing the limits of his autonomy and power. Behind this often lies an unexpressed wish for the impossible, and a bit of magical thinking—"if I can only get over this hurdle, I'll be okay and all will be as it was before."

Anticipating and preparing for threatening new experiences help the elder imaginatively ready himself for what is to come. This is also a good time for encouraging reminiscence and mourning of past periods of better functioning. Understanding that the present behavior is an effort to hold on to what is no longer follows naturally from reminiscence. It often precedes acceptance of a changed self and the need to find new ways of doing things.

In Supervision

For the practitioner, bargaining can most often be deduced from attitude and behavior. The worker will be preoccupied with one case above all others in the caseload, or overidentify with the older person in family interactions. As with the older person in the bargaining stage, the issue is one of control; but it is expressed differently: "If I just do enough for this client she will be able to . . . or not have to."

The supervisory task is to help the worker identify the unrecognized wish behind her overactivity and accept the limits of her power. For the worker, as with the older person, confronting her lack of control over the ultimate outcome of the situation is painful. The realization that there are circumstances beyond one's control is hard to acknowledge.

By the time workers have reached the bargaining stage, they are usually responsive to a supervisor who suggests that they look at their own motivations. They may be embarrassed when confronted with their own rescue fantasies; but are usually thankful for an opportunity for discussion. Workers who care the most are usually the ones most affected and the supervisor should validate the investment in client well-being before challenging overzealous behavior.

Anger and Sadness

Anger and sadness are closely linked emotions in old age. They share the same root: feelings of helplessness and hopelessness. At times they coexist, with one masquerading as the other. They are the most common responses of worker and client to loss and dependence.

Anger

In Practice. Anger is marked by feelings of helplessness—not always directly expressed. Finding fault with one homemaker after another may be an older woman's expression of mourning that she is no longer able to care for her own needs. Client anger may also be expressed passively, such as forgetting appointments or failing to follow through on agreed-upon tasks. Dissatisfaction with services and criticism of her helping efforts cut deep with the case manager or direct care worker who is trying so hard yet can never please.

The novice worker often responds defensively to client outbursts, pointing out the falsity of each criticism or trying to quiet the client with reassurance. Such interventions lead to client-worker power struggles and a breakdown of the helping relationship.

To avoid a power struggle, the worker has to first identify the source of the elder's anger—which may or may not be the matter under discussion. If the worker is to blame, she needs to admit it. If she is not, she needs to be helped not to personalize anger which arises from the client's own feelings of loss. Finally, she must allow a safe place and sufficient time for the client to express negative feelings that are not easily tolerated by family and friends.

For the client who expresses anger passively, a gentle confrontation is often in order. Pointing out the disparity between what the client had said and what he did can invite the client to express negative feelings directly.

In Supervision. Helping the worker handle client's anger means understanding how hard it is to have one's helping efforts spurned. Often the worker responds with anger on her own. This may be directed toward the agency or toward herself. When the worker's anger is justifiably directed toward an unresponsive service system, the supervisor can teach skills in working with the environment: advocacy, brokering, and mediating with one's own and other systems. (Interns will benefit from process recording and analysis of their work with other helping professions.)

When the worker personalizes an older person's anger, the supervisor can help her maintain focus on client assessment. Understanding the possible causes of the behavior is the first step toward helping the worker help the client air his grievances more productively and appropriately. In a more difficult case, the worker may need help in identifying and accepting her own dysfunctional interactive patterns with the client that may have spawned the dispute.

Sometimes, of course, the worker's anger at agency, supervisor, or the entire service system may not be a reflection of client anger at all, but the outcome of his own deep dissatisfaction at receiving too much interference, or too little support, or perceived lack of progress with clients, or personal problems unrelated to the job.

As the worker's task is to move the angry elder from reactive expressions of anger to proactive means of control, the supervisor can help move the worker from reactive anger at the system to proactive advocacy efforts on the elder's behalf and on his own.

Sadness

In Practice. Elders suffering from a clinical depression will experience a variety of symptoms requiring psychiatric assessment and intervention. However, for many ill and disabled older clients, there is a pervasive sadness and passivity that may not reach the level of a psychiatric diagnosis but is nonetheless troubling. The sad elder may view his situation as "all or nothing." If he cannot be restored to who he was before, what is the use of trying?

The elder's sense of dependency and helplessness mirrors that of early life. Now, as then, he must borrow strength from the bond with a caring, supportive figure. This role is appropriately filled by the case manager who needs to recognize when referral for a psychiatric evaluation is necessary and the direct care worker who needs to learn the words and actions that are most useful with an elder who expresses hopelessness and negativity.

In Supervision. As the older person may become hopeless and negative in the face of irreplaceable losses, workers often suffer a paralysis of thought and action when confronted with the multiple losses and prognosis of many elderly clients. How can the worker provide hope when she has none?

The supervisor can be most helpful here in sharing her own professional experiences. For example, a paralyzed, wheelchair-bound woman in a nursing home will remain in that state regardless of first-rate nursing or social work intervention. However, finding activities she can enjoy and working on improved relations with her family can lead to improved psychosocial functioning and a higher quality of life for her. Selective sharing of the supervisor's own positive experiences and best-case scenarios can help the worker imagine the positive and the hopeful.

As the elder must adjust self-expectations to meet the reality of her losses, the worker needs to grasp the concept that work with the aged often involves maintenance of existing strengths rather than dramatic improvements. In fact, incremental changes may be all that are achieved. The supervisor who finds satisfaction in the incremental growth of the worker can demonstrate this attitude through role modeling.

Negotiating the Balance Between Dependence and Independence

In Practice

It is hard to imagine a situation in which an ill or disabled elder cannot exercise some measure of choice and control over his life. It may be as simple as choosing his clothes for the day (or whether to get dressed at all) or favoring one position in bed over another. Independence of choice does not depend on the cognitive, physical, or sensory abilities of the client; but it does depend on the ability of the worker to recognize and honor the client's wishes.

For many older people, there are large areas in which they can continue to exist independently—although dispirited by their ailments or passively accepting the direction of others they may cease to try. The inexperienced worker may perceive giving up as "realistic," or she may focus on the specific request for help, bypassing the broad-based assessment that would reveal whether the client were indeed functioning at the optimum level possible given his disabilities. Many deficits are correctable, at least in part, by introducing aids, training, and minor changes in lifestyle. All of these factors must be explored before concluding that the client must accept his limitations.

When current functioning is the best possible, it is the time to introduce life-enhancing activities to replace those that are irretrievably lost. This is a good time for the worker to contribute her knowledge of community programs and opportunities.

Sometimes the client is able to negotiate the dependence/independence balance after a long period of worker investment. The relationship is so solid and gratifying on both sides that it is difficult for the worker to terminate. The worker's task here is to review with the client their work together to date, and to establish if there are future goals to be met. Even if there is no immediate need for an ongoing relationship, a period of less frequent contact is a useful prelude to termination allowing the client a chance to manage his own affairs while still assured of the worker's involvement.

In Supervision

When a worker has successfully negotiated the balance between dependence and independence in her work with ill and disabled older clients, the supervisor will experience many emotions; relief that she can move on to more problematic workers, pride in a job well done, vacillating between holding on and letting go.

As with the client, the contract can involve a renegotiating of the frequency and content of the relationship to allow for increased worker autonomy—always with the opportunity for consultation and support. A worker's gains can also be consolidated by placing her in an advisory, and—in time—supervisory capacity with newer workers.

Chapter 4

Styles of Learning and Teaching

Each worker has an individual style of learning and helping. In an effort to conceptualize these styles, many educators have created typologies. All agree that it is rare to find anyone exhibiting a pure type. More commonly, individuals are prone to one form of learning and use the others to a lesser degree. Identification of learning styles is more than an academic exercise; it leads directly into the selection of supervisory approaches and strategies for case managers, interns, and direct care workers.

LEARNING STYLES

There are three basic learning styles. We identify them as the intuitive, the intellectual, and the practical. Each can be recognized by the worker's dominant mode of response to a situation. Which of the following descriptions most closely resembles your own style and that of those you supervise?

Mrs. W. reports that severe arthritic pain kept her from attending her great grandson's first birthday party. The intuitive learner would most likely respond with how difficult it must have been to miss the event. The intellectual learner would be more apt to ask specific questions about the symptoms and medical treatment. The practical learner would probably move quickly into a discussion of adaptive equipment and transportation that would be useful in the future.

Obviously, any or all of the above responses could be appropriate given the assessment of Mrs. W. and her situation. It is the frequency of one kind of response, regardless of the circumstances, that identifies the dominant mode of learning. Let us look at the hallmark of each type.

Gerontological Supervision
© 2008 by The Haworth Press, Taylor & Francis Group. All rights reserved.
doi:10.1300/5153_04

The Intuitive Learner

The intuitive learner leads with her senses. She is empathic with the emotions of her elderly clients. Empathy, in this sense, is clearly separate from altruism. Most case managers, interns, and direct care workers are motivated by their feeling *for* the client and desire to be helpful. The intuitive learner goes one step beyond: she feels *with* the client.

This situation can have positive and negative consequences. As the intuitive learner is so attuned to the feelings of others, she says what others wish to hear. She engages a wide range of clients easily. She generally has a "third ear" for the communications of her clients—hearing the unspoken that lies beneath the surface of their words. This empathy will sometimes lead her to unquestioningly accept the client's point of view on all matters. She is more often accepting than judgmental of the various maladaptive ways that her clients may live their lives. She is particularly able with elders who have sensory or cognitive impairments and is often creative in her assessments and interventions.

Judy was a middle-aged woman who entered social work after working many years as a freelance artist. She had never set foot in a nursing home before nor had she read anything about the aged. Mr. B., an eighty-seven-year-old man with advanced Alzheimer's disease had been admitted three days earlier. Floor staff could not handle his agitation. She sat with him a bit and recognized that the focus of his distress centered upon three abstract paintings hanging on the walls of his room. Hearing from the family of his prior interest in horse racing, she removed the pictures and replaced them with magazine illustrations of equestrian pastimes. He quieted almost immediately.

Linda was a home care attendant for Mrs. P. who, aphasic following a severe stroke, could only communicate with cries and moans. Within minutes Linda could differentiate and respond to her moods and wishes.

Sometimes the intuitive learner may so join with the client that she is unable to visualize, much less express, a differing point of view. When the elder says she will not accept a homemaker because she fears theft, she takes on the client's fear. When the elder is angry with his son, she too becomes angry.

The intuitive learner will take risks, not all of which have successful outcomes. However, her genuine feeling for the client usually sees her through the worst blunders. Another characteristic of the intuitive learner is that she is frequently in "over her head" and does not recognize it. As she is so comfortable exploring feelings, she may inadvertently open up an issue with the client that she does not know how to handle. In an extreme case, she may empathize so much with a depressed, suicidal elder that she cannot imagine an alternative reality.

The supervisor of an intuitive learner will need to help her make conscious what is now done naturally. With the case manager or intern, she will label techniques and build in the theoretical underpinnings of practice so that the learner can identify and control her responses. Intuitive direct care workers are valued precisely because of the sympathy and concern they feel for the plight of those they serve. However, this can easily lead to overidentification and burnout. What is more, it is often difficult for the direct care worker to recognize that this is a problem or to ask for help. In these cases, the supervisor may need to take the initiative—beginning with a discussion of the many ways in which the client's life experiences and needs differ from the provider's own.

The Intellectual Learner

As the intuitive learner leads with her senses, the intellectual learner leads with her mind. She wants to anticipate and prepare for encounters with elders. She believes that the more she knows beforehand, the better the result.

She is often strong in observational and analytic skills but may be slow to put her insights into practice. She is more comfortable exploring facts than feelings. When intellectually oriented case managers or interns interview the client, they prefer a multiple-choice tool. If they do not have one, they tend toward a question and answer format.

Intellectual learners are particularly interested in the workings of the organizations, such as the chain of command. Direct care workers who learn intellectually will want specific instructions as to how to fulfill their job descriptions. The case manager or intern who is interested in clinical work is drawn to theoretical approaches and practice readings. She welcomes bibliographies. She delights in the discussion of personality dynamics—examples of which she may see in her own caseload. When the direct care worker is an intellectual learner, she will also be quick to bring failures of the care plan or system to the supervisor's attention. Intellectual learners are often reluctant to assume any work responsibilities until they have anticipated the pitfalls.

Avery, a case manager, was assigned ten cases in her first week of employment at a home care agency. A week later she had not had one contact. The supervisor thought that hiring her had been a poor decision until she learned that Avery had used the time to read every piece of literature about the agency, its referral sources, and through all of the client records. She had also discussed the cases with other members of the interdisciplinary staff. For each elder and homemaker, Avery had drawn up a list of possible issues and responses. Feeling in control, she was able to move into the work quickly in the second week.

Susan who was known as a first-rate direct care worker balked at taking on a new case and her supervisor was puzzled. It took a bit of questioning for Susan to admit that she had never known a blind person and was afraid that she would say or do the wrong thing. With some help anticipating the situations she might encounter and guidelines on how to handle them, she was able to move comfortably into the new assignment.

The supervisor of the intellectual learner will need to help her gain awareness of how her feelings affect her work with clients. As this learner is better able to integrate intellectual and emotional ways of understanding, she will gain comfort in dealing with emotionally charged material and ambiguous situations.

The Practical Learner

If we continue with the analogy of leading with the senses and the mind, the practical learner leads with her hands. She is guided by a desire to make things better and seeks every opportunity to perform a concrete service. As elderly clients present many concrete service needs, those who serve them have plenty to keep them occupied. When the learner is a practical case manager or intern, she will have up-to-date procedural information and foster good contacts in entitlement agencies. The practical direct care worker will be effective in organizing her time and tasks.

The practical learner is less attuned to the problems of clients for which there is no immediate solution. Unlike the intuitive learner who feels the client's pain as her own or the intellectual learner who asks where the pain comes from, the practical learner may not recognize the pain at all.

As she approaches life in a pragmatic fashion, she may expect the same from elders and families. She may become puzzled or angry when they do not act in ways that she thinks are in their best interests.

> Priscilla, the case manager, told Mr. J.'s son exactly the documentation he would need to apply for Medicaid for his father and coached him on every step in the process. When she called to check on the application, she was shocked to learn that he had not even made an appointment. Although he had expressed regret about being unable to support his father, she could not take in the emotional impact of this information and its probable effect on his behavior.

> Bill, a home health aide, prided himself on work with paralyzed clients. He worked out a good system for helping Mr. T. to eat when they were alone together and could not imagine why the client refused his help when others were present.

The practical learner, like the intellectual learner, is more comfortable with facts than with feelings. However, while the intellectual learner's goal is understanding the problem better, the practical learner's goal is uncovering a solution. In her desire to bring about change quickly, the case manager or intern tends to take over more of the work than she needs to. In her desire to get the job done, the direct care worker may not recognize the disabled elder's need to appear self-reliant. If the practical learner is unable to provide a solution, she is usually ready with advice and suggestions to the client on how he should manage his problems. His lack of follow-through is a source of annoyance.

The practical learner learns primarily from trial and error. Over time she realizes that some interventions are usually effective and so broadens their application to different cases. She recognizes that other interventions do not work and gradually stops using them.

The particular challenge of supervising a practical learner lies in appreciating and supporting the very real skills required to carry out a concrete task, while demanding a more reflective level of practice. The worker needs to become more reflective abut the meanings and consequences of her behavior and that of her clients. With increased self-awareness, she will be better able to enable clients to think through solutions and to act on their own behalf.

Again, it is rare to find a worker who fits only one of the above categories. The more able the worker, the more all three styles are used appropriately. However, identifying the worker's *primary* learning style helps the supervisor decide what style of teaching will be most effective.

TEACHING STYLES

There are three major types of teaching that are utilized within the supervisory relationship: collaborative discussion, didactic instruction, and experiential exercises.

Each method has its virtues. Each method complements the others. The proportion of any one type of teaching depends upon the type of learner and the issue to be taught.

Collaborative Discussion

Collaborative discussion is the mutual give-and-take of conversation. It is the most frequently used teaching technique. In educational supervision, it is initiated by the supervisor to explore the intern's thinking on a case. In administrative supervision and consultation, it is often initiated by the worker who has identified the problem for discussion. Exploring, drawing analogies, generalizing, and partializing are all forms of collaborative discussion that can be useful in modeling how to approach a problem through logical analysis.

Exploring

The supervisor should ask rather than assume why a particular intervention or idea governed the worker. Sometimes good intentions underlie an insensitive response or ineffective action. An intern or beginning worker may need support for a good intention before being able to accept criticism for an intervention.

Sally, a home care attendant, asked a depressed man if he would take a whole bottle of pills if he had them. The supervisor was appalled but restrained herself and asked Sally what she had been thinking of at that moment. Sally said that she had heard somewhere that if depressed people talked about suicide they were less likely to do it. This alerted the supervisor to a training need for all the direct care workers as well as an issue with which this worker needed help.

Drawing Analogies

Drawing analogies between the client's situation and the learner's own life and difficulties in practice can promote greater understanding.

Jeff, an on-site social worker, complained that he was frequently called upon to intervene in arguments between residents of the assisted living facility. They were all old and sick. Why couldn't they just get along? The supervisor pointed out that congregate living situations—dormitories and senior residences—had similarities. Were there any people in Jeff's dormitory that he had differences with? How did he handle them?

Generalizing

Generalizing is a way in which the supervisor organizes elder's attitudes or behaviors into a pattern. In so doing, she helps the worker make links between theory and practice.

Tasheka, a case manager, reported that Ms. J. slept poorly and found no pleasure in visits from her neighbors that she used to enjoy. The supervisor suggested that these might be symptoms of a clinical depression and suggested that they look together to see whether the client exhibits some of the other criteria of that condition before deciding what to do next.

Generalizing can also be useful in helping the worker make connections from case to case.

Maria, a home attendant, complained that a new client with severe vision loss was afraid to go outdoors with her. The supervisor reminded her of other cases where she had gained the trust and confidence of clients and asked how she did it. Maria then remembered a few phrases and interventions she had used that worked. (Often surface differences between cases—such as the gender or health problems of the client—obscure the similarities in their situations.)

Partializing

Partializing involves breaking a problem into manageable parts.

June, a case manager, was overwhelmed with the multiple problems of a new case and had no idea where to begin. The supervisor suggested that they list the problems the K. sisters had since the death of their caregiving niece: they are mourning her loss, unable to manage household chores or finances. The landlord is threatening eviction. The nephew is advocating nursing home placement. She then asked: What is the most urgent need? What is the most amenable to the interventions of our agency? What is better referred outside?

In collaborative discussion, it is wise to begin discussion in a manner that accents strengths and mitigates deficits of the worker's learning style.

Let us imagine supervision on the case of Ms. G. an eighty-seven-year-old community resident for whom a nursing home is being discussed. We will envision how the collaborative discussion might evolve with three case managers exhibiting the learning styles previously identified.

Ally, an intuitive learner, laments that Ms. G. will surely die if she has to go into a nursing home. The supervisor recognizes that Ally is expressing her own feelings about placement. Overidentifying with Ms. G., Ally needs help separating her thoughts and feelings from those of her clients. The supervisor helps Ally look at differences between her life experiences, current situation, and personality and that of Ms. G. before they begin to discuss the plan.

Juan, an intellectual learner, announces that Ms. G. will not survive long in the nursing home. The supervisor knows that Juan has read about the high mortality rate in the first few months after nursing home admission. He needs help integrating this information with the case at hand. She points out that studies have shown that the highest risk is posed to those who are most ill on admission. Adequate preparation and involvement of the elder in the planning minimizes the risks. The supervisor also shares a few clinical experiences of her own nursing home admissions. She is careful to include her emotional reactions to the placement. In this way, she urges Juan to consider his feelings and those of Ms. G. Then, they discuss how he and the client can work together on the move.

Amy, a practical learner, comes into supervision and says she is ready to take on a new case since her client, Ms. G. is all set to enter the nursing home. As Amy takes pride in her ability to maintain frail elders in the community, she has interpreted the placement as a professional failure. She has "written off" Ms. G., unaware of the emotional support she can offer in the transition period. The supervisor helps Amy review her work with Ms. G., pointing out what she has done and the circumstances that were beyond her control.

They discuss how Ms. G.'s daily routine will be different in the nursing home, and how Amy can prepare her for the changes.

Collaborative discussion benefits all learners to a certain degree. It forms a useful bridge between didactic instruction and experiential exercises. It also models how the worker can most effectively interact with clients. However, collaborative discussion can easily digress into social chatter unless the supervisor maintains control and focus.

Didactic Teaching

Didactic teaching is what one typically associates with the teaching role, familiar to both supervisor and worker from their years in the educational system. Didactic teaching consists of straight information giving. The supervisor gives assigned readings or oral presentations relating to basic knowledge skills, and tasks to be done in each case.

As it is very comfortable, many supervisors use it exclusively. It feels good to impart wisdom. Most workers feel that they are indeed "getting something" when they emerge from a session with a notepad full of instructions. Used extensively, however, didactic teaching blocks off the worker's participation in and responsibility for her own learning.

Paradoxically, it is the intellectual learner, the one who likes didactic instruction the most, who benefits the least. She will revel in the information and theories that are given (and inflate the ego of the supervisor by respect for all she knows). The tip-off that it is not working is the difficulty this worker might have translating knowledge into practice. Week after week, she experiences the same problems in her cases. Understanding does not inexorably lead to doing.

For the intellectual learner, didactic teaching is best followed by experiential exercises. This is a necessary prelude to deciding what to do next on that case. The practical learner also expects and takes well to didactic teaching if it is informational. Explanations of theory or personality dynamics are best illustrated with case examples. The intuitive learner can benefit most from didactic teaching. It is illuminating for her to get an outside perspective on her feelings—to recognize that there is a body of knowledge and skills that validates her impressions and provides a structured way to offer help.

The limits of supervisory time—and the value of having it spent in mutual exchange rather than a lecture—dictate that additional ways of imparting information be used. When doing so, it is important that the supervisor balance ongoing support with the expectation that the supervisee bears responsibility for her own learning.

Judy, a social work intern, typically entered supervision with a list of questions: Does Mr. V. have Alzheimer's disease? Is it safe for Ms. I. to have cataract surgery? The supervisor soon found herself using up most of the supervisory hour giving lectures. Soon realizing that she was the only one doing any work, and that her well-intentioned efforts were actually precluding the intern's participation in her own learning, the supervisor changed course. She suggested that Judy look up information for herself and check it out against the client's situations before their next meeting. Then they would work together on deciding upon an appropriate intervention.

Experiential Exercises

Experiential exercises are a form of reentering past interventions or anticipating future interventions between worker and client. Role-play and line by line reading of recording are two methods of this approach. While line by line reading can be used effectively with workers, it depends upon the presence of detailed process recording that is usually done only by interns.

Most supervisors and workers shy away from experiential exercises. When drawn into them, they begin with great reluctance. Workers are often afraid that they will say the wrong thing and be judged incompetent, or they will complain that an artificial simulation of a contact can never reflect the real thing. Supervisors are often afraid that their own responses might not be up to par and they will be judged as less than competent by their workers. However, the usefulness of this approach becomes readily apparent once initial doubts are overcome.

Role-Play

Role-play can be done with the supervisor playing the worker and the worker playing the client, or the reverse. When the supervisor plays the worker, she does more than model good responses or provide the words the worker may be lacking. She listens carefully to the way the worker portrays his client and for client feelings that have not emerged in the worker's recordings or oral presentations.

When Lisa played Mrs. W. with an exaggerated shining tone, it was immediately evident to both supervisor and worker that Lisa's negative feelings about the client were influencing the interaction.

When the supervisor plays the client, she allows the worker an opportunity to try out various interventions. It is useful here to begin by asking the worker for her worst case scenario. Often the worker is afraid to broach a difficult subject or to explore deeper for fear that the elder will become angry and break off contact, or become sad and start to cry. Simply voicing these fears is helpful. When the worker has rehearsed responding to anger and sadness, the real situation becomes easier to risk.

Line by Line

Process recording is an educational tool used in the educational supervision of social workers. It consists of a narrative, sequential written report of an interview with particular attention to the words and actions of client and worker. Although the writing is too time consuming to universally recommend it to graduate professionals, it can be usefully assigned when a worker is having trouble with a client or collateral contact and the source of the difficulty cannot readily be ascertained.

Line by line reading is done of a section of the process recording in which the difficulty was experienced. The worker reads aloud, stopping after each interaction to recollect his feelings and thoughts at the moment. Interventions are then examined, critiqued, and replayed. Finally, the worker anticipates how he might respond to a similar situation the next time around.

John returned to the point in the process when he changed the subject after Ms. P. started to complain of urinary incontinence. He recognized his embarrassment. He also realized that she was trying to resolve whether or not to have surgery and needed to discuss the pros and cons with him. With the supervisor, he figured out a variety of appropriate responses for discussing intimate matters with older female clients.

Experiential exercises are useful for practical learners who are especially adept at role-playing the client. Often, their greatest fear is of client anger or rejection if they do not accomplish some concrete task.

Intuitive workers are also helped by role-playing encounters from both client and worker points of view—demanding that they separate their feelings from those of the client at each step of the process.

Experiential exercises are initially difficult for the intellectual learner. She may have trouble remembering the interaction of an interview and is usually clearer about her analysis of a situation than of what actually happened. She may falter over the choice of words, fearful of saying the wrong thing, even in a simulated interview. It is more productive, at first, for the intellectual learner to role-play the client and the supervisor to play the worker. In so doing, the supervisor can demonstrate interviewing techniques while the worker views the situation from the client's perspective.

Part II:
Supervising Social Workers/ Case Managers— Practice Skills

Chapter 5

The Interview

Gerontological practice is based on the one-to-one contact between the older person and the case manager or social worker. It is through this intimate contact—"the interview"—that all other functions are delivered. Comprehensive assessments and workable case plans are based on what information is gathered and what relationship is formed within these meetings. No matter where the interview takes place, it requires a number of skills on the part of the worker; skills that the supervisor can help her workers master.

TUNING IN/ANTICIPATORY EMPATHY

Entering the world of an ill or disabled elder is, for many case managers, like entering a foreign country. While they may "feel for" the client (sympathy for his condition and a desire to help), it is difficult

Gerontological Supervision
© 2008 by The Haworth Press, Taylor & Francis Group. All rights reserved.
doi:10.1300/5153_05

to "feel with" the client (understand the meaning that his condition holds for him). Tuning in is an anticipatory step that the supervisor and worker can take together. Looking at the face sheet or intake information that already exists on the case, the supervisor can ask the worker to anticipate how the client might feel about his situation and the upcoming appointment.

When John read that eighty-five-year-old Mr. P. had been a practicing attorney until his heart attack a month ago, he realized that continuance of a profession for so long meant that Mr. P. had been highly functioning and committed to work, and that slowing down would have had a devastating affect on his self-image.

Tuning in will also arouse curiosity on the part of the worker—curiosity that will suggest important areas to explore with the client.

John wondered what had happened to Mr. P.'s clients—was there unfinished business that might be weighing on his mind? He also noted that Mrs. P., a second wife, was sixty-four years old and employed part-time. He wondered about how the heart attack had affected the marriage, whether there were adult children from the first marriage who were involved, and about home care eligibility and financing.

Anticipatory empathy also prepares the worker to imagine how his visit may be experienced by clients who have difficulties seeing, hearing, or understanding, or those who have no such problems but are unaccustomed to having a stranger enter their homes. Asking permission to remove distractions (such as turning off a television set) or to reconfigure the seating (such as moving a chair to where he can be seen and heard most clearly by the client) may feel intrusive to the case manager, if he thinks of it at all.

Speaking clearly, simply, and slowly is an aid to communication, but it can be patronizing if exaggerated. Each case manager has to develop her own style and recognize where common or colloquial speech will need to be modified in a practice setting.

When Stacy reported on an interview with a client about problems she was having with her home health aide, she said: "What's the trouble with you guys?" Understanding that Stacy had made a common error and not wanting to embarrass her, the supervisor treated the matter lightly by asking "Since the client and aide were both women, why did you call them guys?"

Stacy laughed. "Yeah, it's just an expression I use all the time. I never realized that it must have sounded strange to her."

ENGAGEMENT

The social work injunction to "start where the client is" is particularly valuable when working with ill and disabled elders for whom a warm-up period is often a necessary prelude to getting down to business.

Forming a working relationship with the older person is the first and most important task of the case manager. If a worker is anxious about how she will be accepted by a new client (or how she will be able to fulfill the agency mandate to gather pages of information on the older person's functioning) she is liable to introduce herself and her affiliation briefly and then move right into the business at hand. The pace and tone of this encounter is often too rapid for an elder who meets few people outside his daily orbit and needs a longer period of acclimation. Taking more time to "get acquainted" by commenting on the family pictures or belongings on display—even talk of the weather—is not idle chat, but gives the older person a chance to adjust herself to the worker's presence. It also gives the worker a chance to observe the client's cognitive and sensory level, and prepare her to guide her interview accordingly.

Engagement is a process through which the older person develops positive feelings toward the case manager and the fact that they will be working together. If the older person is lonely and confused, she may welcome a new person into her life though unclear as to why she is there.

Halle told her supervisor: "Mrs. L. welcomed me enthusiastically and barely listened as I identified myself as the social worker sent by the home health agency. She eagerly tried to help me with my coat and offered me a piece of fruit."

The issue for supervision in this example is what constitutes engagement. Is Mrs. L. clear about the role of a home care case manager? Is she truly so receptive when the worker addresses her problems with incontinence? More than other populations, older people will reach out for company, but this is not engagement. At the same time, the prevalence of physical and/or mental impairments can make a simple introduction problematic.

Sammy told his supervisor: Mrs. N. has been in the nursing home for three months and is paralyzed and speech impaired. I introduced myself and explained why I was there. Mrs. N. smiled and said "yes, yes, yes." I felt good because it sounded like she wanted help, but she suddenly began to cry and clutched my hand frantically.

In this instance, the supervisor provided basic information about aphasia and how to determine the client's level of comprehension. As with hearing loss, creative interventions and a high tolerance for frustration are necessary to develop a helping relationship.

Often older people are referred to agencies because someone close to them notices a decline in their functioning. Yet the client resists this interpretation. In fact, reference to problems can be perceived as threatening. At the same time, the case manager needs a point of entry.

Mrs. Z. was referred for social services by the home care nurse because she was depressed. She insisted that she needed help only with getting Medicaid reinstated. She bristled at the word "depression" insisting she was not crazy. In supervision, the worker asked how she could contract with the client to accept a psychiatric evaluation. The idea of initially working on the concrete needs while establishing a relationship and assessing mental status was comfortable for the worker. This plan made the contract clear and honest, but allowed for changes in the future.

In other cases, it is the worker rather than the client who has difficulty in putting the problem into words.

Mr. P. was identified as a good case for a social work intern by the floor team because he had experienced a severe heart attack and the death of a roommate within a month's time after which he became angry and demanding with staff. It was hoped that contact with a social worker would improve his behavior. Jane, the intern asked for help in engaging this involuntary client. She feared that he would identify her with the other staff whom he saw as always trying to make him do something he did not want to do. After a role-play with the supervisor in which she put herself in the client's shoes and tried to imagine his feelings, Jane decided upon her approach. She began by acknowledging that two serious incidents had happened to Mr. P. in a very short time and imagined how difficult that could be for him. He said "You wouldn't believe it" and went on to describe the night of his heart attack. At the end of the interview, they agreed that there was more to talk about before he could get "used to the changes."

With the cognitively impaired, the dilemma is even greater since the building of a relationship will not necessarily make the problem clearer to the client.

Mr. H. an eighty-nine-year-old homebound elder sometimes thought Millie, the case manager, was his nurse. At other times, he thought she was his daughter. It was hard for Millie to get beyond the problem of mistaken identity to see her role with him. In supervision, she and the supervisor looked at the help she could offer—listening and responding to his reactions of the moment, observing his functioning, monitoring the relationship with the home care attendant, acting as a bridge to the nurse on the team and interpreting the agency's role to the family. Knowing there was something she could "do" gave Millie the role she sought. In time, she appreciated that her very presence and interest was a service to the client whether he recognized her or not.

Case managers new to the field of aging are initially nonplussed by clients suffering from dementia. They may discount anything the client says as being irrational and therefore meaningless. The supervisor can help the worker recognize the difference between intellectual and emotional functioning. Even in cases of severe mental impairment, the feelings remain intact. Anger, fear, pleasure, anxiety, and sorrow are common human feelings. It is to these feelings that the worker must relate.

ACTIVE LISTENING/OBSERVATION

Case managers may become frustrated when older clients persist in talking about matters unrelated to the purpose of their meeting. Elders may tell the same story the worker has heard many times before, ask personal questions, make social conversation, or return to issues the worker thought were already resolved.

Changing the subject is rarely effective. What is more, it deprives the worker of valuable assessment information. The client may be lonely and hungry for any human connection or too confused to recognize the worker's role, but he is communicating something important. It is up to the worker to find out what it is.

Active listening (what has also been called "listening with the third ear") is paying attention to the communication that lies beneath the spoken word. Observation is taking in all the nonverbal ways that people convey their emotions. The supervisor might help the worker uncover the underlying content and link it to the assessment.

Mrs. J., confined to a wheelchair after a hip fracture, had been an award-winning real estate saleswoman and insisted on showing Daniel the certificates she had to prove it. Not only did she do this every visit, but the showing was accompanied by the same stories of how her boss could never get over her abilities. Daniel complained to the supervisor that all this time spent "bragging about the past" was getting in the way of Mrs. J. discussing problems in the present. When the supervisor asked Daniel why he thought these stories were important to Mrs. J., he thought for a while and then said "because she wants me to know that she was once important?" The supervisor asked why Daniel thought that she was doing this. After a pause, he said "she isn't important now?" Together they looked at the many meanings of the "bragging," and how he might respond.

EXPRESSED EMPATHY

Ill and disabled older people—particularly those who are isolated and hungry for recognition—often share more of their previous lives or current problems than the case manager wants to, or feels she needs to hear. Impatient to get on to what she sees as the purpose of the meeting, the worker may let these remarks pass without comment or quickly refocus.

The worker who is afraid to risk expression of her own feelings in the interview may hide behind a professional facade. Yet, comments that indicate that the worker recognizes and appreciates the message behind the words are important; helping the client feel "heard" and appreciated for the individual he is.

Reading over a record in which the only notation about children was "Ms. J.'s only child, a daughter, committed suicide at the age of twenty" the supervisor wondered how Jodie, the case manager, felt hearing that information. Jodie said "awful . . . it was so sad . . . and I could tell by the way she said it that she thinks of it all the time." The supervisor asked if she had expressed any of this to the client, Jodie said "I just went on to the next question. I didn't want to make her feel any worse." The supervisor wondered if this effort to spare the client may actually have made her feel that her pain was not understood. Together she and Jodie looked at empathic comments that could be made in these or other situations.

The action-oriented agenda of case management often leads workers to disregard problems about which they can do nothing. They may have trouble simply acknowledging a client's distress. Risking a few personal responses ("that sounds difficult," "that is so sad," or "how disappointed you must have been") not only brings the client closer to them, but also brings them closer to their shared humanity.

EXPLORATION OF FACTS AND FEELINGS

The best way to learn about a client's view of his problem is to ask him. Such an obvious statement should not be necessary, but it is. Some workers give greater credence to the reports of other health care providers and family members than to the views of the client himself. This is most often the case when the client is cognitively impaired, physically very frail, or has difficulty in hearing and communicating. Exploration uncovers the many factors involved in a client's presenting problem in order to understand it in depth. Most importantly, exploration identifies what aspects of the client's story to investigate further as well as when and how to do so.

Case managers are usually more comfortable exploring facts than feelings; partly because they have the agency form to guide them. It is easier to ask how often the client receives help from his children than how he feels about it; to obtain the names and contact information of his health care providers than how he feels about the care he receives from them. Yet such information is an important indicator of the help he needs and his readiness to receive it.

Feelings arise from facts. The worker need not parrot "how do you feel about that?" but can help the client expand on his story in a way that will make his feelings self-evident.

The supervisor noted that Jane's client assessments all looked the same—a summary of concrete needs. Even though there was a space for her to write "Impressions"—no individualizing comments differentiated one client from another. Jane understood that she was supposed to find out about the client's feelings about receiving help but was unsure how to go about it. The supervisor suggested a few open-ended phrases that could open up discussion ("Tell me more about that," or "What happened the last time you got together") after each question was answered. Jane was surprised to see that the feelings the client had about the situation emerged with the story. What is more, the expanded answer to one question actually answered two or three others further down on the questionnaire.

The elderly client has, of course, a longer story than other clients. The worker needs to learn how to elicit information and how to focus while still offering an empathic ear to all other information the client wants to share. Issues related to dependence, isolation, loss, and illness always need exploration.

The supervisor commented to Ellen that Mrs. L. often says that she never wants to be a burden to her son, and wondered what exactly she meant. Ellen said that Mrs. L. was very independent. The supervisor agreed but wanted to get beyond that summarizing statement. She suggested a role-play with Ellen as Mrs. L. She asked Mrs. L. to tell her about her son. As Mrs. L., Ellen expressed a fear of "bothering" him. She also talked about her daughter-in-law and past strains in the relationship. From this exercise, Ellen began to think of issues for further exploration.

Information about a client's capacity for adaptation and coping is often embedded in stories from the past—as are dormant client strengths that may be mobilized to deal with current situations. The worker with no background in the meaning of life review or reminiscence may discount such stories or cut them off.

The key to teaching workers the skill of exploration is in arousing their curiosity. Younger clients or clients presenting problems closer to those of their workers naturally inspire greater curiosity. The concerns of the elderly are often assumed to be one-dimensional and concrete. The supervisor can help the worker appreciate the complexity and the challenge.

Mattie reported that Ms. P., who lived in a large house, told her that she had a tenant, another older woman who never seemed to be around during their visits. At the same time, Ms. P. referred often to this woman's activities and opinions. The supervisor said it sounded odd that the tenant had such sway over Ms. P., yet never showed herself to the worker. She encouraged the worker to make a point of involving the tenant—and found that she was not a tenant at all, but Ms. P.'s partner of many years and that both women feared that their relationship would not be accepted by the agency. With this information, many puzzling aspects of the case management situation suddenly made sense, could be discussed openly and resolved.

Sometimes beginning workers fear exploration because it is seen as "prying." This belief is true in work with other age groups, but it is especially true in workers who have been brought up to "respect" the aged and interpret respect as not questioning anything they say. If this appears to be an issue, the supervisor can help to show the difference between the personal and the professional self. The analogy of a physician may be helpful; that is, she must ask the elder to disrobe and raise questions that would not be permissible in ordinary social relationships.

The case manager needs to look for the meaning behind nonverbal behavior and repetition of thoughts or incidents, which signal that a more complex meaning is hidden in the words.

CONTRACTING

The final step of the initial client interview is contracting. Contracting is a verbal agreement between client and case manager about what they will be working on together and what their respective roles will be. (Calling it an "agreement" is usually more appropriate with older clients.) The contract—or agreement—may also include the time frame of future contacts, and next steps each of them will take before meeting again. In some cases, it is necessary to restate the contract at each meeting and/or be satisfied when the client cannot participate fully.

Jo, social work intern, came to her supervisor in distress. She was supposed to write a paper about "contracting" with her first client but Mrs. N. was demented and could not participate. The supervisor asked why Mrs. N. thought she was coming to see her, Jo replied "I'm the nice person who likes to help old people." They both agreed that this was a sufficient contract.

With clients who are cognitively intact, recontracting is often indicated. This can take place when the situation changes, or done at periodic intervals to make sure that the client and worker stay on track.

Chapter 6

Assessment, Case Planning, Ongoing Work, and Termination

ASSESSMENT

Assessment is not an accumulation of facts about the older client. It is an interpretation of those facts; a sifting through that establishes their relative importance and interaction. Most assessment forms contain information about the medical, psychological, social, and cultural background of the client. The wealth of material makes it essential that the worker be able to discern patterns and determine relevance.

Case managers and social workers need to become familiar with the chronic health problems, acute illnesses, and common accidents of the elders whom they serve and the usual treatments for these conditions. This information—familiar to practitioners who have been trained as nurses or other health care providers—may seem overwhelming to a case manager with no medical background. Agency-based training and handouts provide basic knowledge; but if it is not immediately applicable to the worker's caseload it is apt to be forgotten.

More useful is the expectation that the worker will learn about the health conditions of each of her clients. The first client with arthritis, or heart failure, or a hip fracture, or multi-infarct dementia should prompt reference to a medical dictionary, *Merck Manual, Physicians' Desk Reference,* handouts from various organizations as well as Web-based search and consultations with health professionals on the team. Over time and experience with many clients suffering from the same problems, the case manager will develop a knowledge base sufficient to identify health care problems and refer them appropriately.

Gerontological Supervision
© 2008 by The Haworth Press, Taylor & Francis Group. All rights reserved.
doi:10.1300/5153_06

To help in understanding psychological content, the supervisor can sharpen the worker's ability to listen to themes as well as content.

> Sarah was frustrated that Mrs. K. always criticized her efforts. The supervisor suggested that they look together at all that was known about Mrs. K. The facts that she had been orphaned at an early age, had an unhappy marriage, complained about her care at the hospital, had a daughter who never provided good meals, and a son who never visited were in the record, they had never before been linked together. When they were, Sarah realized that feeling uncared for and having unmet needs were basic themes in Mrs. K.'s life that were enacted with everyone she met.

Social Supports

Social and cultural information should not be interpreted too quickly. The fact that an older woman has a daughter who lives nearby does not mean that she is a source of "social support." An older man who appears alone in the world may have a neighborhood shopkeeper who looks after his needs. An individual of a certain racial or ethnic background does not necessarily prefer a certain diet or method of address. Easy assumptions often turn out to be wrong.

> · The supervisor assigned Keesha, a recent immigrant from Africa, to work with an African-American client. Keesha began the interview by calling the woman "Mama." The client was irate "I'm not your Mama. I don't even know you!" Keesha was upset and puzzled as addressing the elders in her town by this name was a sign of respect. This encounter made Keesha doubt her ability to work with clients whose culture and worldview were so different from her own. Helping her sort out similarities and differences between the life experiences of her clients and herself, the supervisor helped Keesha recognize her strengths and avoid future pitfalls.

CASE PLANNING

Planning is not a linking of care needs in Column A with services in Column B—or hooking the client into the system. It is a process of making the system work for the client by selecting services appropriate to his individual situation. Careful attention must be paid to informal and formal supports, either existing or potential, that can be utilized on the elder's behalf. Foremost, is salient information about the family (the family of origin as well as the family of mid and late life). Family history impacts heavily on the elderly person's life situation and his feelings about it. Information about neighbors, friends, and agencies involved in the elder's care round out the picture.

Separating Fact from Inference

Beginning workers often have difficulty in separating data from opinion, and fact from inference. It is critical that they learn to do so. Accomplishment of this task in written form may require many attempts. The supervisor can begin by helping the worker back up her opinions with factual examples.

Maryanne returned from her first home visit and announced to the supervisor that the client belonged in a nursing home. The supervisor responded that the mission of the agency was to keep elders in the community as long as possible. She would have done better if she had asked the worker what she had observed that led to that conclusion—and so missed the opportunity for a discussion of assessment.

Long-Term and Short-Term Goals

The establishment of long-term and short-term goals is both the outcome and the purpose of the assessment. Goals are the expected result of the case manager's intervention. The best goals are written in measurable terms, expected time frames, and phrased from the client's point of view. For example, Mrs. J. will find an alternative living arrangement that offers housekeeping services—six months: Mr. W. will accept home health care twenty hours a week—one month. Measurable terms and expected time frames allow the supervisor and worker to monitor progress and revise case plans as necessary. Phrasing from the client's point of view keeps the worker faithful to the client's wishes rather than imposing her own.

It is useful for the supervisor to periodically help the worker reconnect with the goals of a case. Sometimes unforeseen situations arise making it impossible for the client and worker to reach the goals they are mutually contracted for. If this is not the case, analysis of why goals were not met may require reassessment and new goals replace the old.

Mr. Q. was upset about losing Meals-on-Wheels services and angry at the agency for denying it to him. Rather than defending the agency position, Bob led Mr. Q. into a discussion of all that had been achieved in the past six months since service had started: successful completion of physical therapy after a stroke and a restored ability to cook for himself or go out for his meals. As they spoke, Mr. Q. realized that what he missed most of all was the friendships he had developed at the rehab center. Together they set a new goal of participation in an aftercare program.

ONGOING WORK

With the exception of acute care, medical, and psychiatric settings, most agency practice with elders is open-ended—an appropriate modality for a population whose needs often fluctuate. As a consequence, workers may focus their attention on new cases or those in which a crisis is occurring while offering the others periodic monitoring and supportive services. The danger here is that important developments after the initial assessment may be overlooked, or that elder and worker may reach an impasse. When this occurs, the supervisor should help the worker return to the assessment and case plan and reevaluate the intervention strategy.

· Supervisors may believe that little intervention with workers is necessary once a case plan is underway. Yet, as the helping relationship progresses, topics for discussion between the worker and client tend to veer away from immediate needs. Boundaries between professional and personal use of self blur. The worker often has trouble in focusing. It is also during the ongoing phase that the client reflects upon his life and other issues with which he is concerned. For this reason, it is useful for supervisors to periodically review ongoing work with their supervisees.

Focusing

Workers often have difficulty structuring their contacts with older clients. Often they report "the conversation turned to" or "the subject changed" as if they have no responsibility for the direction of the interview. Although the client's free association may be useful in psychoanalytic practice, it is not the model for goal-directed case management, especially with the elderly who have a tendency to digress. Digression may be a way of avoiding a discussion of painful subjects. However, it is often the result of cognitive or sensory impairment, unfamiliarity with the norms of a counseling interview, or social isolation and delight at having someone to talk to. The skill of maintaining focus on the work—without preemptively cutting off important material that initially may sound irrelevant—is difficult to achieve. The worker should use the initial and ongoing assessment as a guide. Above all, the worker must learn and feel comfortable with the words that will shift the client from an unproductive to productive pattern of thought without alienating or angering him.

The supervisor role-played the situation of Mrs. F. with Cynthia. Mrs. F. hung on at the end of every interview and would not let her leave. She suggested phrases the worker might use to leave comfortably. ("In the time we have left, let's. . . ." or "Next time we meet, we can. . . ."). Cynthia also used supervisory help in preparing to focus Mr. Z. who had limited hearing and sight. She learned to touch him on the arm when she wished to interject a comment or change the course of the discussion.

Multiple Losses

While dealing with painful feelings is a hard task for any practitioner, the case manager may feel especially hopeless when confronted with multiple losses.

Jane described to her supervisor how depressed Mrs. C. seemed. Jane remarked that Mrs. C. would start to say something and then stop, saying "what's the point?" The supervisor asked how Jane felt about Mrs. C.'s situation. Jane reluctantly said that Mrs. C. was right—she had little to look forward to; illness and death were all that lay ahead. "So what is the point?" asked the supervisor. Jane talked about her previous job with troubled adolescents, and how there was hope no matter how bad the situation was. The supervisor asked if it felt different with Mrs. C. because she was old. Jane agreed, but soon added that Mrs. C. had more insight and understanding than her previous clients, and recalled illustrative incidents. The supervisor and Jane then discussed how work with Mrs. C. could help her cope better with her daily life.

Case managers often feel so helpless when confronted with the multiple losses of their clients that they quickly move away from discussions of "sad" topics to reminiscences about a time when life was better. Uncomfortable with negative feelings, they may stress the positives that life still holds. The supervisor can help them recognize that talking about a happier time when they were more able is important to many older clients—helping them mourn their losses as well as sharing their life experiences and lessons with an interested younger person.

SPECIAL ISSUES

Reminiscence

Elderly people often enjoy talking about the past, but do not necessarily need the case manager or social worker to help them do so. The worker needs to use reminiscing as a tool rather than as an end in itself. When the worker has identified what the elder's present-day problems are, reminiscence can be directed to a past coping pattern that can be utilized in the present. It can also be directed to long-held attitudes that might be presenting obstacles in the present situation.

Mrs. D., an eighty-five-year-old woman, was a day care member who needed to apply for Medicaid and food stamps. Each time she met with Rita, the case manager, she spoke repeatedly of her need for services, but did not bring in the filled out forms as she had promised to do. The worker was stuck until her supervisor observed that Mrs. D. had survived the Great Depression and wondered if she had received government help at that time. The supervisor suggested that it might be a fruitful area for exploration. When Rita asked Mrs. D. how she and her family survived the 1930s, she heard a compelling story of coping with adversity. Mrs. D. talked contemptuously of those who gave up. The worker then asked if government help felt like "giving up" to her. Mrs. D. responded that she had no choice, but it did. They continued to talk into the next week about the WPA and other subsidy programs. Mrs. D. was then able to submit the documentation and complete the application.

Sexuality

Perhaps no aspect of work with the elderly elicits more discomfort than issues of sexuality. Evidence of an older person's interest in sex, not to mention active participation, is enough to generate embarrassment among those around them, including professional workers.

At the same time, the practitioner needs to look carefully at today's more liberal view of sex in late life. While sexual interest and activity is more acceptable and common for the elderly than it was in decades past, there is still a significant decrease in sexual activity. Discomfort talking about sex is neither uncommon nor surprising in a generation who came of age before the sexual revolution. Often, however, it is the worker who shies away.

Judith, a recent social work graduate who came from an Orthodox Jewish family, took a job in an agency providing mental health services. Counseling Mrs. L., an elderly woman whose husband had died three months earlier, she was dumbfounded when Mrs. L. expressed regret that regular sexual contact was over. In supervision, she and her supervisor discussed Mrs. L.'s artistic background and sexual attitudes that were quite different than Judith's own. At their next meeting, Judith expressed appreciation to Mrs. L. for verbalizing her concerns and suggested that they now work on Mrs. L.'s sense of loss and unmet needs.

Homosexuality among the aged is an issue that often arouses judgmental feelings on the part of supervisors and workers. Although older gay men and lesbian women are usually childless, they often have a support network of friends who function as surrogate family. Older gays and lesbians may have special financial problems because pensions and social security benefits for life partners are not available for them as they would be for a spouse. In addition, many have lived a lifetime of sexual nonacceptance which may foster secretiveness, anger, and anxiety. Supervisors and workers must be sensitive to the unspoken messages of single older people who often present their needs in veiled terms.

Mr. P., a seventy-nine-year-old retired bachelor, attended a day program for the visually impaired elderly. He told everyone that he boarded in a house owned by another man. When this landlord died suddenly he came to the program director asking for help finding another living arrangement. As she explored further, Mr. P. told her how bereft he was. This man had been his "best friend," "psychiatrist," and "brother." As the worker encouraged him to speak more she understood that the deceased "landlord" had been a life partner and recognized the special anguish Mr. P. felt at being unable to grieve publicly. Although Mr. P. eventually told the director that he had lived as a homosexual all his adult life, he asked that she not tell others at the center who "would not understand." This experience raised the director's consciousness to the importance of recognizing and legitimizing nonfamily relationships of her older clients and helping her staff to do so.

End-of-Life Issues

Workers may be two generations younger than their elderly clients and issues of death and dying are far removed from their personal lives. The fact that their clients have already lived beyond normal life expectancy and could die at any time can be frightening to novice practitioners who find discussions of death and dying quite overwhelming. The older person, on the other hand, may bring the subject up frequently, almost casually, in conversation.

As there is so much useful literature on death and dying the supervisor may have to restrain herself from inundating the worker with too much information. Instead, she will want to focus on an understanding of the issues that may arise and of behaviors and attitudes that may accompany them. This method will help the worker understand what the elder is trying to say and respond accordingly.

Mr. S. an eighty-six-year-old childless widower, persisted in asking Lu to check and recheck his burial arrangements with his lawyer. He resisted efforts to talk about his underlying fears. In supervision, Lu was encouraged to drop the focus on Mr. S.'s fear of death and explore his past. In discussing his past, it became apparent that Mrs. S. was the dependable relative in his family who made all the arrangements for everyone. Now there was no one left to arrange things for him after he died. An arrangement with a funeral home for a prepaid funeral lessened his anxiety.

Feelings of helplessness as the elder's life comes to an end are common. These, too, can be worked on in supervision.

When Mrs. N. was hospitalized and near death, Andrea told her supervisor how uncomfortable she felt visiting her. Andrea felt she just sat there while the medical team carried out their procedures. The supervisor asked what Mrs. N. wanted at this point. Andrea thought a while and then said "someone who would be with her, listen to her if she felt like talking, and tell her the truth." Armed with the knowledge that Mrs. N. needed someone who would not deny her present state, Andrea was able to "just sit" with her.

No amount of reading and lectures will make work with the sick and dying easy. These are the most painful and frightening areas for any practitioner. The supervisor who can listen to such difficulties and provide needed support, can make an enormous difference in how the practitioner manages the process.

TERMINATION: CLOSING A CASE

Closing a case is often emotionally painful for client and worker. Ideally, termination is a time when the client has no further need of services. In practice, termination is often more involved with agency dictates, the worker changing her job or the end of an intern experience. It is not uncommon for the worker to experience guilt and anxiety about abandoning the elderly client. As agency resources are often scarce, the worker's perception may be correct. It is likely that the client will receive fewer services when the worker leaves—especially if the worker is an intern. There is never a good time for a worker to terminate. Frail elderly clients are prone to emergencies that inevitably turn up as the worker is ready to broach the subject of his leaving. Of course, the aged have had much experience with loss and have developed coping strategies to adjust to the loss of a significant person. However, the loss also conjures up painful memories.

Supervisors can help workers identify what work has been accomplished during the time of the relationship and role-play ways in which this "case review" can be conducted with the client. This is empowering to the older person who can recognize tasks accomplished and look forward to continuing with a new worker. It is also reassuring to the departing worker who can recognize the lasting effect of his involvement.

At the time of termination, issues of professional boundaries quickly come to the fore. Interns and workers typically experience conflicts about gift giving and continued visiting or letter writing with the older person after their departure. It is helpful in supervision to focus on the end of the professional relationship. Even if the practitioner could visit regularly, the relationship has changed and is no longer the same. As the worker takes in this concept, he can focus on pieces of the relationship and how much of the relationship is involved in work issues. Interns or workers can begin to share this thinking with the client: "Even if I came to visit you, I couldn't help you with changing your health aide." The intern or worker will also begin to understand that visits and other communication will only disappoint the elder as a close relationship cannot usually be sustained.

Assigned readings on the meaning of termination in the therapeutic relationship are helpful. They provide departing staff with a conceptual understanding of the impact of their departure on clients and themselves. The supervisor can follow up by helping the worker anticipate how the news of termination will affect each of his clients. An individualized approach and time table for working it through can then be implemented.

The intern or worker is also terminating with the supervisor. The supervisor's role modeling of how one says good-bye in a professional relationship will underscore the importance of reviewing and coming to terms with the relationship. These actions allow both parties the freedom to move on.

Case closing due to the death of a client is an often unrecognized source of distress to the case manager (as well as other members of the care team—especially the direct care worker). Agency responses are usually limited to the writing of a final note, removal of the client's name from a list of active cases, and the assignment of a new case to fill the gap. Although this efficient process meets administrative needs, it does not begin to address feelings connected with losing a client with whom one has had a bond over time. For many staff there is no place to express their grief. When the situation warrants it, opportunities should be provided for workers to attend funerals, pay condolence calls, and share reminiscences with family members and with co-workers. Staff meetings or group supervision provide excellent opportunities for clients to be remembered—as well as to provide group support and supervisory recognition of one of the most difficult aspects of work with ill or disabled older people.

Chapter 7

Empowerment, Mediation, and Advocacy

BEYOND THE ONE-TO-ONE

Case management with elders is far more than one-to-one encounters with the client. In fact, interventions with others in the client's world often consume most of the worker's time and effort. Loosely united under the heading "systems work" this includes the "informal system" (family, friends, and neighbors) and the "formal system" (other community, health care, and social service providers).

Successful outcomes of these encounters require the case manager to assume different roles and use different skills than called for in her work with elders. A supervisor may suggest that the worker "involve the family," "get in touch with the landlord," or "work with the doctor," assuming that the worker has an understanding of the purpose of these encounters and the skill to carry them out. When the worker fails or "forgets" to follow through, or the encounter is botched, the supervisor knows that it is time to back up, assess the worker's view of her role, and work on skill development.

The worker may have unexpressed reservations because of confusion about what constitutes confidentiality—what legally needs to be communicated to other professionals and what is protected or privileged information. The beginning case manager will also need guidance about the interplay between what is confidential in her work with the elder and what needs to be communicated to the family. Occasionally, she will be misapplying a psychoanalytic model of attention, rather than viewing her work in a systems perspective. Problems of

Gerontological Supervision
© 2008 by The Haworth Press, Taylor & Francis Group. All rights reserved.
doi:10.1300/5153_07

elder functioning that involve other people are more likely to be resolved with those people present. This is a difficult concept to get across with many workers. Bright, otherwise able workers may be intimidated by a brusque physician or an unfriendly nurse and so limit their interventions to areas not involved in another discipline's expertise.

Well-mannered workers may feel that they must take an aggressive stance with other disciplines or providers of help—setting up an adversarial situation where none need exist. When it comes to work with families, an overidentification with the client, and judgments about how partners or adult children "should" feel and act may get in the way of productive interventions.

· This chapter discusses how the supervisor can teach the skills of empowerment, mediation, and advocacy as they apply to work with families and with other health care providers. Underpinning these skills is the understanding that accepting help always involves a trade-off: exchanging a measure of independence for a measure of support. Practice approaches with the older person thus find their parallel in supervisory approaches.

GENERAL ASSUMPTIONS ABOUT DEPENDENCE

Assessment of the specific older person or specific worker in terms of their need and capacity is based on a few general assumptions about the nature of dependence.

1. *Dependence is partial, not total.* However disabled, the older person can do something—even if it is just to raise a finger to indicate yes or no. However inexperienced, the worker can do something—perhaps she can handle concrete matters independently, but has difficulty with emotional content.

2. *Dependence is temporary, not permanent.* The older person's disability curve is not a straight dive downhill any more than the worker's learning curve is a straight upward climb. There are many plateaus, unexpected spurts forward, and disheartening regressions.

3. *Dependence may be in doing, not planning.* There is the apocryphal story of the old woman who said, "Just because I need help crossing the street doesn't mean I don't know where I'm going." This is matched by the worker who understands the purpose of a family conference

and can set it up very well; she just doesn't know what to do with all the people once they get there.

4. *Dependence may be in planning, not doing.* If the older person is asked, "Do you want a homemaker?" and says, "No," that is not self-determination. Older people may lack the information or opportunity to talk through alternatives that are necessary for informed decision making. The worker may be able to follow through on directions, but unable to initiate a plan.

In short, we cannot speak globally of dependence or discuss in general terms how to respond to it. Rather, our assessments of the individual elder or worker situation must specify: Dependent in planning or action? Dependent for how long? Dependent in what ways? What is required is an assessment of dependency in each situation, and choosing a method of doing the work that best meets each need.

SYSTEMS INTERVENTIONS: COMMONALITIES AND DIFFERENCES

Skills of work with the elder's informal and formal system have much in common. The necessity for multiple identification (empathizing with several, often contradictory, views of a problem) and the ability to present one's position in a way that will help others in pursuit of their own goals is primary. This frequently requires a more direct, assertive stance than is usually practiced in the one-to-one therapeutic encounter. Also required is a knowledge base that moves beyond individual psychodynamics to an understanding of systems theory as it applies to family relationships, organizational development, and community organization. Work with collaterals makes professional and personal demands. The worker must be comfortable enough in her role to be challenged—prepared to sometimes "lose" her point, and stay focused on the client situation rather than be distracted by personality conflicts with colleagues. She must also be able to tolerate the ambiguity of unresolved situations and have the patience and skills to work them through. None of this comes naturally, any more than work with clients comes naturally. Workers gain competence from the opportunity to discuss issues of mediation and advocacy in supervision. Through it all, worker and supervisor must decide among three choices "not doing," "doing with," and "doing for."

"Not Doing" Empowerment

Supervisors and workers are constantly presented with situations that require action. Clients and families expect solutions to their problems. Agency administrators expect documented results. Interns must meet the performance criteria set by their school programs. Helping clients, and families act on their own behalf is harder than taking over the work and doing it oneself. Helping workers think through a problem and decide among various approaches to its solution is harder than instructing them as to what to do. What is more, it takes longer. So worker, as well as supervisor, need to believe that helping people help themselves is time well spent.

A refusal to get involved may also be appropriate when the need or request for help is clearly not within the purview of the worker or supervisor. A home health attendant should not be doing heavy housecleaning. A worker need not comply with client demands that she run errands for him. A supervisor need not comply with worker demands that exceed her job responsibilities. However, it is good practice (and good supervisory technique) to avoid the punitive taint of withdrawal from a problematic situation by exploring why needs and requests are unmet and how the client or worker can find alternate means of providing service.

Helping clients and workers mobilize their strengths begins with asking them to reflect upon how they handled similar experiences in the past. It continues with suggesting tools that will help them handle the task in the present, and concludes with assurance of support as they branch out on their own.

Mrs. J. told Kevin of the problems she had in communicating with her doctor. He was always rushed, and she never had her questions answered. She asked that Kevin call the doctor "man-to-man" and find out what she needed to know. Kevin, a beginning worker, was happy to comply. When the supervisor asked him why he rushed to the phone, Kevin responded that he was flattered that Mrs. J. had such confidence in him and wanted to demonstrate his desire and ability to help—especially since so many of Mrs. J.'s problems did not have such an easy solution. When the supervisor suggested that they review all they knew about Mrs. J., Kevin realized that he had not explored sufficiently before rushing to action. Mrs. J. was capable of making her needs clearly known to others and had the skills to do so with the doctor if something else was not getting in the way.

If the worker assesses that the client has the strengths necessary to handle matters on her own, he can work on anticipating and preparing for stressful encounters. Some clients are helped by making lists of questions and concerns in advance of their meetings with health care providers. Other clients are helped by role-play situations with the worker in which they "try out" various approaches. Still other clients need help in organizing their thoughts and can move independently from there on.

The same principle applies to workers. The supervisor empowers workers by helping them reflect on previous cases in which similar situations arose, identifying what strategies were then effective, and asking them to consider how the lessons of the past instance might be applied to the current situation.

The law of parsimony dictates that the least invasive intervention should be tried first. If client or worker need a bit more help, mediation may be the next step.

"Doing With" Mediation

"Doing with" is sharing the work. It fosters control and mastery over what can be done independently and supports what needs the help of another. Each piece of work has many tasks. Qualifying for Medicaid can pose a dozen or more tasks for the elder: assembling documents and making decisions at each stage of the process. The elder will be able to complete some tasks alone. With others he will require the assistance of the case manager, intern, or direct care worker. Similarly, acquiring the skills to see the elder through the Medicaid application encompasses many tasks for the worker. Some of these can best be mastered through didactic teaching, some through reading, and some only through experience. Sometimes a task may not be assigned to one or another but be handled cooperatively. When the worker accompanies the client to the Medicaid interview or doctor's appointment, she is offering support as well as role-modeling ways of handling anxiety-provoking situations. When the supervisor asks the worker how she will prepare the elder for these encounters and helps her consider the pros and cons of various approaches, she is role-modeling how one tries to anticipate the consequences of one's actions.

"Doing with" or mediation is the primary skill in work with families and professional health care providers—each of whom brings needs and resources to the task. For example, family members may have the skills to negotiate a complex system but require direction as to where their efforts will be most effective.

"Doing For" Advocacy

What of the unilateral "doing for" that workers and supervisors continually find themselves pulled into? Is it ever appropriate by itself?

"Doing for" may well be the first case management intervention with the elder when physical or cognitive impairment renders him incapable of a task and there are no friends or relatives to act on his behalf, or when technical agency communication is required. It is also a good point of entry with the suspicious elder who requires tangible proof of the worker's investment before he can trust. Hands-on intervention can provide the nurturing environment in which the chronically dependent elder can function optimally, as well as legitimize the dependency needs of the staunchly self-reliant older person.

"Doing for" is the most comfortable intervention for direct care workers. Helping older people accomplish activities of daily living that they cannot handle alone is, after all, the reason they have been hired. So it is particularly important that those who hold these jobs be helped to identify and support what the elder can continue to do for himself.

"Doing for" may well be appropriate when one is supervising a beginning worker who requires a grounding in information and skills before she can meet her clients with any confidence. "Doing for" is the entitlement of any worker when the demands of the assignment exceed her capacities or when she needs the support of a caring supervisor. "Doing for" needs no apology when used appropriately. It is only destructive when it preempts the elder or worker's own ideas and abilities.

Advocacy is best tried when empowerment and mediation have failed. Mediation validates and recognizes divergent points of view. Advocacy sets up a win-lose situation between the worker and the target of her intervention. The point may be won, but the future relationship may be sacrificed. Members of the interdisciplinary team who suffer a loss of face are less prone to cooperate on succeeding cases. The worker who loses her point suffers a loss of credibility on future issues.

WORK WITH FAMILIES

Supervising work with families often begins by promoting curiosity within the worker. Equally crucial is exploring their attitudes about the role and responsibilities of family members. The expressed wish of an older client not to be a "burden" or of a daughter that her other siblings not be called as "they aren't much help" are often accepted at face value. Exploration may yield more sources of support than initially thought. Once the worker has begun thinking in terms of family with every case, she must make individualized assessments of her clients and develop a method of capturing significant information. (The genogram is a useful tool that can be used with alert elders. A completed genogram orders the family information already known and determines areas requiring further exploration.) After all the involved and potentially involvable family members are identified, it is helpful to explore the worker's perception of each one's stake in the care plan for the elder. Finding commonalities in conflictual situations are crucial to the success of family work with the elderly. These techniques can be practiced within the supervisory conference.

Johanna, director of a day care program for older people with dementia, told her supervisor about the problem she was having with two sisters—one who volunteered to pay for nursing home placement for her mother, and the other who was equally committed to keeping her in the community. As she spoke, the supervisor realized that Johanna was disapproving of the working daughter who she saw as "pushing" placement and was siding with the "stay at home Mom" daughter as the older woman's savior. In fact, she had set up a power struggle where none needed to exist. The supervisor decided to ask Johanna for the underlying content beneath the spoken messages. The working daughter's message was that if her mother was in a nursing home, she would feel less worried if she had to go out of town and was willing to pay for that peace of mind. The housewife daughter's message was that she would feel more secure about her mother if she could maintain control over her diet by bringing over foods she had prepared. When commonalities in the message were underscored—both daughters were found to be concerned and wishing to contribute what they can—the stage was set for a productive family conference.

(A variation on this theme is an experiential exercise in which the worker is asked to pretend that she is each family member and voice their concerns about the central issue.)

While raising worker self-awareness prior to meeting with families is essential, a successful encounter is not assured. Often the worker may feel overwhelmed: by individual family members who are perceived as powerful authority figures or simply by conducting a group interview. She may be confused as to where her primary allegiance lies—setting up a false dichotomy such as elder or family. She may fear antagonizing one family member if she plans a conference to include others of whom he has spoken with disapproval. For these reasons, the supervisor can never assume that the worker with a sound assessment can move easily into a family intervention.

Preparation for the family meeting should center upon as accurate a prediction as possible of what might occur. Surprisingly, it does not matter if this prediction is borne out in the ensuing contact. The worker who is well prepared for several contingencies has developed a sense of confidence and flexibility that can serve her well when the unexpected arises.

Janie, a twenty-three-year-old first-year social work intern in a hospital's neurological unit had to meet with her ninety-two-year-old client's two nieces and their husbands. They had come from out of town to discuss care plans after Ms. W. suffered a severely disabling stroke. Janie was overwhelmed because all four people she was to meet were middle-aged professional people; two with administrative positions in health agencies. The supervisor helped Janie anticipate this family's need for full information about options before making a decision. Marshalling all the resources and the pros and cons of each, helped Janie feel more secure. She also realized that she lacked sufficient understanding of the prognosis and sought clarification from the staff physician. She secured his availability to speak to the family if necessary. The supervisor advised Janie to concentrate on the messages beneath the positions and to reach for negatives before assuming consensus. Most important, Janie was reminded that she was not responsible for the decision; that was with the family. She was, however, responsible for ensuring the best process possible. The interview turned out differently than had been anticipated. One niece began by saying that she had washed her hands of all responsibility, to the shock and dismay of her sister. The men sat helplessly quiet. Janie had to switch gears immediately, abandoning all that she had prepared. However, she proved well able to mediate the family conflicts and emerge with a viable plan for the aunt. When the supervisor complimented her later, Janie remarked that she remembered that it was the family's job to come up with a plan and her job to give them the information and facilitate their decision.

Whenever possible, elders should be present in any family meeting in which their fate is decided. Families may need time alone first to plan how to orchestrate this participation. In cases, as the one portrayed above, the elder may be too incapacitated to participate in a family meeting. The worker, then, often needs to be reminded that it is her responsibility to speak for the elder's point of view and report back to the elder (with or without the family) what has transpired.

Supervisory time spent going over the intricacies of one such encounter is often enough. However, there should be the expectation that the worker will be able to translate the principles to similar situations. Readings are especially helpful as an adjunct to preparation for family encounters. As with most reading assigned in supervision, this should be practical rather than theoretical. Interview transcripts, audiovisuals, or practice texts that focus on case examples are most helpful.

WORK WITH OTHER CARE PROVIDERS

The worker in a community or long-term care setting must learn to see the facility through the client's eyes—and understand the client's relationship to each of the disciplines involved. Complaints about care are common. Considering two possibilities simultaneously—that there may be a concrete problem and that the complaints may indicate an underlying emotional issue—is one of the first lessons that the beginning worker learns.

Mr. R., a nursing home resident, repeatedly complained to his new social worker, Michael, about long waits for care and rude treatment by nursing assistants. Eager to resolve the situation Michael set up a meeting between Mr. R. and the charge nurse. At the meeting, to Michael's chagrin, Mr. R. denied any complaints and assured the nurse he had no problems at all. The supervisor asked Michael what he thought was behind the denial. Michael suggested a fear of reprisal. The supervisor agreed, and also suggested that, some complaints mask feelings of despair and loneliness. How could Michael find out what was really going on? Relieved of his embarrassment and newly curious about Mr. R., Michael was ready to participate in a role-play to improve his skill in exploration. He also decided to do more observation on the floor.

Smaller community agencies may not employ other disciplines, and teaching the skills of collaborative work is harder. When trying to contact a professional health care provider, the worker does not have the opportunity for goodwill built up through a shared work environment. The status differential between case managers and physicians can be intimidating. Identifying with the need of the other party is a useful strategy that can be anticipated in supervision.

The need for mediation between elders and the formal system often comes into play in cases of noncompliance with health care directives.

> Mrs. L., an obese eighty-seven-year-old diabetic widow, confessed to Gennie, the case manager, that she frequently cheats on her diet. Her justification: "What else do I have in life to enjoy?" The fact that she had pledged Gennie not to tell her doctor only became known to the supervisor when the client became an emergency admission to the hospital in a diabetic coma, and the worker came to her in the throes of guilt. Upon exploration, Gennie said that since she had agreed with her client that she was entitled to pleasure in food, she felt it wrong to argue with her.

This explanation tipped the supervisor off to the dearth of intervention options that the worker had at her disposal, and the necessity of teaching skills of mediation.

> Knowing that a successful aftercare plan for Mrs. L. would require the case manager's collaboration with the doctor and the hospital nutritionist, the supervisor explored her feelings about speaking to other health care professionals and found that Gennie frequently felt inadequate in understanding medical terms and did not know how to respond when told that people were too busy to speak to her. Her first assignment was reading material on diabetes published for the layperson. Her supervisor assured her that she needed no more medical knowledge to converse effectively. Second, the supervisor gave her some phrases to use when she felt "brushed off" by other professionals. For example, "I know from the past that Mrs. L. will be unable to follow your diabetic regimen without further discussion with you. As you are busy now could you please tell me what would be a more convenient time for me to speak with you?" While it wasn't important, or even desirable, that the worker repeat these words verbatim, possessing them gave her a sense of comfort and direction.

Part III:
Supervising Social Workers/ Case Managers— Administrative Issues

Chapter 8

The Organizational Context

Supervision consists of three functions: administration, education, and support. In an ideal world, the supervisor who is responsible for keeping statistics, insuring compliance with agency mandates, and monitoring worker productivity is also engaged in advancing staff development and offering workers support with their difficult caseloads. In practice, the administrative function often overshadows the others. Restoring a rightful balance depends on understanding the organization and how to work within its possibilities and constraints.

This chapter addresses organization variables as they affect the supervisor's role as "middle management."

AGENCY SIZE AND AUSPICES

The potential for the full exercise of the supervisory role depends, in large part, on the size of the agency. Size affects the collegial relationships open to supervisor and workers. A large agency offers the

Gerontological Supervision
© 2008 by The Haworth Press, Taylor & Francis Group. All rights reserved.
doi:10.1300/5153_08

support of numbers in advocating for client causes and worker rights—a potential that is not present in a smaller setting. At the same time, larger staff numbers often result in bureaucratic difficulties.

The auspices of the agency are also significant. A public setting or a setting dependent on government funds typically has the most bureaucratic regulations. These agencies are required to implement social policy through a variety of procedures and with extensive documentation. They will have the least opportunity for worker autonomy in task accomplishment.

In settings dependent on public funds, the worker can anticipate layers of bureaucracy, each with limited authority. Change is usually slow. At the same time, directives from the top can change rapidly. Service is determined by fiscal regulations. For example, reimbursement for service to the elderly may not recognize the need to work with family members. Or policy may allow for only a certain number of visits in a fiscal year regardless of needs. In the public sector, workers often feel they are functioning as double agents—balancing client service and gatekeeping functions. It is difficult, though not impossible, to influence this system, as political considerations are usually primary motivations in establishing and implementing service.

Nursing homes and home care agencies are commonly proprietary organizations where the need to make a profit is primary and service is geared in that direction. Often agencies directed toward making profit provide good care. However, for the social worker, providing a softer, less easily measured service, ethical dilemmas can emerge quickly. As a supervisor, one must be alert to maintain professional standards of practice. Paraprofessional workers with little training are most frequently found in settings operated under proprietary auspices. In these cases, the supervisor is usually a consultant, hired on an hourly basis to fill mandated government requirements.

The private sector in gerontology is most often filled by Geriatric Care Managers in small (frequently one-person) operations. These managers charge on a fee-for-service basis.

Voluntary agencies are most compatible with helping professions and gerontological practice. Although often governed by federal/state regulations and funded by public monies, a voluntary agency has an established mission to serve a target population. The presence of a Board of Directors and discretionary funds raised through development efforts allow for services that are not available in less-endowed settings.

In the voluntary sector, policy can change or be modified through assessment of needs, as well as fiscal constraints or change in government regulation. An employee typically has access to a smaller chain of command. (In many agencies, any employee has access to the Executive Director.) All of this means that a supervisor in a voluntary agency has the means to promote improved service or a change in policy. Life is not easy or always rewarding in a voluntary agency; however, possibilities for providing better service in a more benevolent setting are much greater than in public or proprietary settings.

Resources available to gerontological workers are tied to auspices and funding sources. The public sector often has the fewest resources with workers balancing client service and gatekeeping functions.

THE SUPERVISOR AS "MIDDLE MANAGEMENT"

The supervisor may feel torn between her responsibility to her workers and responsibility to upper management. Feedback from other staff is always useful in assessing a worker's practice. However, the supervisor is in the best position to determine how the worker is practicing. She will put the feedback from other disciplines into a context.

The agency administrator always praised Mark for his work and value to the agency. The supervisor was aware of Mark's skills, but also of his tendency to ingratiate himself with authority. She communicated the positive feedback and discussed authority issues with Mark.

Often situations require that the supervisor define the role and method of case managers. Nonsocial work staff often wants immediate solutions from the social worker. Social workers may overstep their bounds in assessing nursing issues. So it is incumbent on the supervisor to negotiate and clarify expertise and roles. He will hopefully modify unrealistic expectations and remind staff of the limits of each profession. Such intervention also helps staff to feel validated and supported.

All supervisory intervention models practice. The impact of the supervisor on the system will have a trickle-down effect on the workers. If she is good at the job, the supervisor's use of self will be reflected in the good practice of her supervisees. As a middle-management employee, the supervisor is close enough to the hands-on experience to understand the clients' needs. She also has enough exposure to the administrative issues to understand the agency's needs and limitations. This unique position offers many opportunities for improvements in service delivery.

ORGANIZATIONAL CHANGE

To effect organizational change, the supervisor must consider the importance of the issue, the resources available, and the possibility of successful outcome. Opportunities to empower the client population are also important and must be addressed, as long as the supervisor recognizes the need for all parties to participate in the process.

The day care administrator regretfully announced that he must cut back the lunch program. All participants in the center were upset. At spontaneous meetings, elders suggested petitions and calling the press as strategies to counteract the plan. The social worker, being identified primarily with the clients, perceived the cutback as an indication of the administrator's lack of caring. The supervisor, understanding the current budget constraints and seeing the potential for enormous problems, worked to defuse the situation. She suggested that the social worker help the members determine a course of action in addition to petitions. She alerted the administrator of the participants' anger and the possibility of a petition. She reminded him that social action was psychologically beneficial for the participants although she agreed it was hard "on us." She encouraged and supported the social worker. However, she also reminded her that the problem might not be resolved in the clients' favor. As the social worker began to see the issue as a process, she was able to work more productively with the group. At the same time the supervisor continued discussion with the administrator. In so doing, the supervisor computed the cost of lunch and persuaded the administrator to present a plan which would allow for lunch at a small fee. The social worker, meanwhile, primed the group for a negotiated settlement. At a large meeting, the administrator's plan was greeted with applause and cheers.

The issue in this example is a conflict between the perspective of workers allied with their clients and administrative decisions that appear to be in conflict with clients' well-being. It is the most common kind of problem the supervisor encounters. The supervisor must think through the range of possible interventions as well as their consequences. She thus speaks for the client while accommodating the administrative needs. Helping the social worker to mediate rather than advocate is primary, as is engaging the administrator in understanding clients' needs for control.

Organizational change requires skill in influencing the key policy-makers in an agency. Although any good case manager will easily identify many unmet needs, resources are limited. Every agency chooses to serve one category of need, while another equally deserving area is not addressed. As an initial step, the supervisor assesses the feasibility of change.

A supervisor at a YMCA Senior Center noted the workers' concerns about the frail elderly who could no longer come in for programs. She decided to develop a program to be presented to the administration. In her plan, one of the social workers would move into a housing complex for the elderly one afternoon a week for social programs. She also contacted an agency that provided in-home counseling for the elderly. She worked out a direct referral system for clients who needed individual counseling.

In this example, the supervisor broadened the agency's scope by providing the same service on a different site. This solution is a relatively simple, inexpensive way of offering service to more people who need it. The supervisor also worked out a mechanism to provide the individual counseling through another agency.

Having to say "no" to an elderly person in need is always difficult for a worker. The administrative supervisor must appreciate these feelings, but also provide an understanding of the larger system. An elderly client at risk in the community, with no family or friends, may have to move to the top of a waiting list of a community service agency. The supervisor must intervene to accomplish this goal. On the other hand, a Christmas dinner for participants in a day care program is a fine idea that may not be possible in a small agency because of cost or need for sanitary kitchen facilities. The supervisor's role in this instance is to interpret the obstacles to the workers and help them look for outside resources.

RECORDING

For the professional worker, recording is an agency requirement rather than a supervisory one. The particulars of recording depend on agency needs and outside funding requirements. The supervisor should monitor recording for promptness and appropriate content. It is not uncommon for the worker to make recording low priority. Paperwork seldom feels significant in the helping process. The supervisor must believe, and demand, that timely recording can and must be a priority.

Recording provides the agency with documentation of its services. It also affords other staff an understanding of the client's needs and the worker's interventions and plans. The ability to do summary recording or a chart note is difficult for many workers to achieve. It requires a level of conceptualization and synthesis different from that needed to record recollections of an interview in process. It is useful for the supervisor to have models or outlines—such as the following—as a guide.

> Mrs. L.'s situation is currently stable. She continues to receive assistance from a home attendant who also does shopping and cooking. She appears increasingly anxious about her son's job transfer even though he will not be relocating. Continued exploration has not revealed any reason for heightened anxiety. Plan: To interview Mrs. L. with her son to further explore his transfer and her concerns. Psychiatric consultation if anxiety reaction continues.
>
> Jane Willis, MSW

* * *

> During this period, ninety-nine-year-old, wheelchair-bound Mrs. O., whose diagnoses include dementia, osteoarthritis, functional paraparesis, myocardial infarction, and cataracts, remained medically stable. At a team meeting on January 22, 2006, she was noted to be unable to walk due to contractures and was at risk for skin breakdown. As a result of her dementia, she can be verbally disruptive, screaming at other residents and agitated at times. She is treated with Haldol for this condition. In general, Mrs. O. can be observed sitting in her wheelchair, obviously disoriented and often appearing detached from her environment. She has the tendency to mumble to herself, sometimes calling out, but her speech is usually hard to understand. As a result, verbal communication is difficult. Mrs. O.'s brother is in frequent contact. He inquires about community services and responds to supportive counseling. He visits his sister often and is a reliable family member. Plan: Show interest and support to Mrs. O through brief individual contacts. Refer brother for assistance with concrete services or counseling

to a social worker. Continue to monitor Mrs. O.'s overall functioning with the interdisciplinary team. As previously noted, discharge planning is not possible. Review as needed.

Timothy Lerner, RN

EVALUATIONS

Evaluations are part of working life. A written evaluation representing each year of the worker's service is the ideal. Although most agencies meet the standard of yearly evaluations, few have a written document. More typically, the evaluation is a checkoff list and may or may not have room for written comments. Personalized comments, differentiating the worker's strengths and struggles from those who share her job description, should always be added.

Case managers should expect that evaluation is an ongoing, mutual process. When discussion and feedback on all aspects of their work is an integral part of the supervisory relationship, the written document should not come as a surprise. The content area will depend on the setting and the particulars of the job, but there are also standard areas of practice that cross agency lines.

Employee: Christine Thomas

Employed: 11/20/05

Evaluation: 11/01/06

Ms. Thomas was employed as a case manager in November of last year. She is a beginning social worker with experience as a teaching assistant. She came to the agency highly motivated to provide service to the elderly. Ms. Thomas has good communication skills evidenced by her ability to work effectively with her team and seek consultation with other disciplines about her clients. She is also sensitive to the needs of the elderly, and assesses and plans for psychosocial interventions very effectively. Providing and understanding concrete services is a new experience for her. She is often frustrated with the slow responsiveness of the system and needs supervisory direction to help mobilize resources. This is an area of continued work. Ms. Thomas has good relationships with her colleagues and is friendly and outgoing. However, difficulties with less responsive staff members are also evident, and a pattern of intervention problems in difficult systems has emerged.

Ms. Thomas is a reliable employee who is on time and completed required recordings and statistics in a timely manner. She is active in staff meetings and volunteered to be present at a staff seminar during the year.

She is overall a highly satisfactory employee. Goals for the year are:

Learn eligibility requirements for Medicaid, SSI, and other entitlements;

Develop skills in negotiating systems;

Develop alternative interventions when frustrated by unresponsive resources;

Examine relationships in the agency and develop more effective interventions.

As the employee evaluation is best seen as a "work in progress"—an interim report that points the way toward future professional development—it is important that it provides goals to strive toward and a framework within which this can be achieved.

Chapter 9

Staff Development

In gerontology, ongoing supervision is of particular importance. There is much expertise about the aging which must be learned on the job. Students completing social work or nursing programs have often had no formal course work in the field. They often possess only a superficial understanding of the psychosocial issues faced by ill or disabled older people or the range of possible interventions. Moreover, the problems of this client group have so many dimensions that the beginning worker needs supervisory assistance to partialize and prioritize what must be done. The more experienced worker may be able to handle complex situations independently but still benefit from consultation on difficult cases and staff learning opportunities that broaden and deepen her understanding—preparing her to someday undertake supervisory responsibilities herself. For all levels of worker, the supervisory relationship provides support, knowledge, and an opportunity for self-understanding—all factors instrumental in preventing burnout.

INDIVIDUAL SUPERVISION

An "open door" policy of one-to-one supervision is increasingly the norm in case management agencies. While this is a necessary response to the crisis situations often faced by the worker (and the need for immediate advice), it is insufficient to meet the case manager's long-range need for professional development.

Administrative supervision addresses the use of agency resources (including the skills of its workers). How can these resources be best allocated? Supervision of even an inexperienced worker is different

Gerontological Supervision
© 2008 by The Haworth Press, Taylor & Francis Group. All rights reserved.
doi:10.1300/5153_09

from supervision of an intern. In the supervision of an intern, the focus is on learning. What knowledge and skills did the intern gain from the experience? While education is important in administrative supervision, the focus is more on outcome. How did the worker's interventions help the client?

Owing to time constraints, most administrative supervision is based on the verbal accounts of the worker—with greatest attention paid to new cases, complex situations, or problems involving agency systems. Apart from those situations, the issues raised depend largely on what the worker perceives as an issue or concern. The supervisor thus needs to be alert to what is and is not raised by the worker.

Andrew's supervisor noted that supervisory sessions over the past several weeks had consisted of a series of questions about tasks and issues related to forms. When questioned, Andrew said that the job required a lot of detail. When the supervisor pressed about some of the more clinically oriented situations, he became defensive. When she noted that there had been several recent emergencies in his caseload and wondered how he felt about them, Andrew quieted down and volunteered that he was overwhelmed, upset, and exhausted.

Often the overwhelmed or irritated worker is not responding to job pressures; rather, she may lack the necessary clinical skills to meet client needs.

Joan is a social worker with two years of post-master's experience in an Employee Assistance Program. She complained bitterly about the time that speaking to families took away from her work with nursing home residents. She particularly resented the demands of one "manipulative" daughter who kept detaining her on her rounds with complaints about service. The supervisor recognized that while Joan was effective with residents and staff, she needed more knowledge and skills to work with family members.

A differential assessment of the supervisee is the key to a productive relationship. Even though there is less teaching with a professional worker, the process is similar to that with an intern. The supervisor starts with worker concerns and builds upon them. As the primary purpose of administrative supervision is accountability for delivery of agency service, the supervisor directs the worker in the use of time and assessment of needs.

A worker's attention will most likely be reactive to the most problematic and demanding cases—and, frequently, conflicts about how to intervene with demanding clients.

Anne, a social worker at a rehabilitation center, asked her supervisor what she should do in the case of Mrs. C. As they spoke about it, the supervisor saw a flicker of annoyance on Anne's face. When questioned, Anne expressed resentment and anger at Mrs. C.'s unending demands. She also explained that "limit setting" did not work because refusing to respond each time Mrs. C. called made her angry with the unit staff. "No way out?" said the supervisor. Anne laughed. They discussed Mrs. C. and together developed a sense of why she was so demanding and untrusting. The supervisor also suggested that Mrs. C. sensed Anne's exasperation and dislike. Together they agreed that shorter, regular appointments might lessen the client's demands and Anne's unproductive reaction. They then talked about staff reactions and worked on interpreting Mrs. C.'s behavior and engaging other staff to promote a consistent care plan.

The beginning case manager often needs help in making the transition from intern to worker.

Wendy had been an excellent intern who was hired by her field placement agency after graduation. She was thorough in assessments and explored every possibility before determining a course of intervention. In her first job, she continued to function the same way and put in hours of overtime. Discussing these issues with Wendy, the supervisor realized that coming to grips with a vastly expanded caseload—and an inability to prioritize—was the problem. This became an issue for future work.

CONSULTATION

At the other end of the supervisory scale is the highly experienced worker. As the purpose of administrative supervision is accountability, ongoing oversight continues to be necessary. Yet, the time for independent practice has to come at some point in a practitioner's career. The supervisor and the worker should mutually set a goal for the time when supervision can be consultation. Supervisor and worker do not always agree at what point a greater degree of independence has arrived. However, the ongoing evaluation of practice moves toward this goal. The worker who is ready to move toward consultation will keep the supervisor apprised of cases and problems. This is crucial in cases that contain possible ethical violations, abuse, legal problems, or liability issues for the agency.

The worker who has reached the point of consultation should also be expected to recognize and ask for help in problems where she is losing her professional perspective.

Joanne a longtime agency employee who also had a part-time private practice, requested a consultation on the case of Mr. K. She began by saying that she was growing anxious each time she had to meet with Mr. K. and needed some time to discuss the case. As she and the supervisor looked at past and current contacts with Mr. K., Joanne realized that she was so identified with Mr. K. that she had taken on his feelings of being abandoned by his son. The consultation ended with Joanne deciding to bring Mr. K. and his son together for a discussion of what each expected from their relationship.

Even the most experienced social worker needs a forum to talk through some of the difficult problems she confronts daily. Overidentification with an appealing client, anger at a demanding one, or frustration at an unresponsive system are all common human reactions. The supervisor can be twenty years younger with half the experience of the senior worker, but can still be helpful if she understands her role. She provides an arena to discuss, identify, and resolve problems interfering with the worker's practice.

STAFF MEETINGS

Most agencies provide learning opportunities in addition to individual supervision. The most common are staff meetings. Information is shared at staff meetings and discussion can also include administrative issues of general concern. One often leads to another.

The supervisor needs to distinguish between what practice issues are best addressed in individual supervision and what are best addressed in the group. Assessing a client's need for an escort to a doctor's appointment is an issue for the supervisory conference. The need for escorts in the population in general belongs in a staff meeting. Staff meetings are often used by workers to express service problems. Sometimes these complaints can be usefully translated into group training opportunities. At the same time, the supervisor must also ensure that worker's complaints are not masking practice problems.

As the supervisor explored Jose's complaints about the services available for Mrs. M., she became aware that Jose's complaints were similar to Mrs. M.'s complaints to him. When this was pointed out to him, Jose was able to see that he was projecting his own anger at the client onto the agency. Other workers were then able to see that they too were picking up and passing on client attitudes.

In an agency that uses conferences or rounds, this kind of example could be used as the focal point of discussion of a common practice problem. When workers recognize that their human responses are understandable and not personal failings they benefit themselves and others struggling with the same frustrations. Rounds should also focus on successful cases. Examining good work reinforces practice strengths and identification of practice skills that may be used elsewhere.

CASE CONFERENCES

Supervisors should seek a balance of case presentations by reaching out for the ideas and practice problems of staff. It is also useful to balance presentations among disciplines and ensure that different skill sets are identified. If the supervisor carries a caseload, it can be useful for her to present her own work. Workers will be able to see that practice struggles continue as a part of professional life, and her presentation style can serve as a model for theirs. Larger agencies often have the resources for more advanced learning. A large social work department may have a speaker address a significant issue. Such a department might also participate in interdisciplinary learning situations. Hospitals and large nursing homes might organize grand rounds for all disciplines. They might also invite an informed professional to address relevant issues in aging.

CONTINUING EDUCATION

Regular opportunities to participate in learning situations, such as conferences and continuing education workshops, outside of the agencies should be encouraged. Workers need to learn of new developments in their field and need to advance professionally. They also need to interact with other professionals beyond the confines of their own agencies. Opportunities for growth and learning keep morale high and provide the agency with personnel capable of providing higher quality service.

The administrative supervisor will recognize that performance expectations differ by discipline and that interdisciplinary collaboration is key. A social worker will be expected to have strong communication and listening skills. A nurse will need to have enough expertise in this area to know when to call in the social worker. Similarly, the social worker needs to have enough clinical knowledge about common medical symptoms to know when to contact a nursing colleague. Both will have to meet the administrative requirements of the agency, be able to prioritize and handle all assigned work in a timely and professional way.

GROUP SUPERVISION

In large agencies, group supervision or peer supervision may be used in addition to—or as substitute for—some sessions of individual supervision. The supervisory assessment of specific strengths and deficits of the setting should be considered in the assessment of each worker's learning and practice needs. (A single worker in a setting will need more opportunities for impromptu meetings, e-mail, or phone contact with the supervisor. Such contacts buttress and reenforce professional identification.)

Group supervision for case managers can be a highly effective way of monitoring practice and using resources judiciously. Meeting with a group of supervisees, rather than meeting individually, is obviously a time saver. In community and long-term care settings, every moment of time is precious, and any opportunity to save time and allocate resources differently is significant. However, time is only one positive factor of group supervision. Case managers potentially come from different professions and have different skills. The group modality offers a fine opportunity for staff to learn from each other. All disciplines have stereotypes and some stereotypes have a basis in fact. Typically, social workers deride nurses for their rigidity and dependence on paper compliance. In return, nurses characterize social workers as "bleeding hearts" focused on process rather than outcomes. Ultimately, case managers have to learn from each other and learn how to use each other's skills effectively. Group supervision is the ideal format to foster this important learning.

In small agencies, two or three case managers can reap the benefits of being seen as a "group." This need not involve extra supervisory time. The supervisor can experiment with paring one-half hour from each individual's supervision and use it for meeting her workers together weekly or biweekly. In addition to learning the skills of another discipline, groups allow for peer learning and support.

Groups also offer a forum for supervisees to challenge the supervisor. As there is safety in numbers, individuals who would hesitate to articulate concerns individually are more likely to raise "uncomfortable" issues in a group setting—often alerting the supervisor to staff issues and concerns of which she was previously unaware. Supervisors also learn more about their supervisees in a group, how they relate to each other, including how they interact with others.

Group supervision needs planning and an agenda. The time allotted may also be shared with a staff meeting (another time saver). In that case, the agenda might begin with discussion of a policy change and plans for implementation. The discussion could then continue with discussion of cases that would be affected by the policy change, and also include discussion of cases reflecting typical current problems. Depending on the issue, several people might present brief case scenarios, or the focus might be on one problem case.

A skilled, confident supervisor will use group supervision as an opportunity to model leadership and learning. As group facilitator, the supervisor's task is encouraging the sharing of ideas, clarifying and restating significant points, focusing the discussion, and summarizing salient ideas to move the discussion forward.

Group supervision is also an excellent forum for a supervisor to identify and help supervisees discuss feelings that they all experience, but fear to express.

Linda, supervisor in a home care agency, met with her six case managers in monthly group supervision. Brian presented the case of a client who had lost her apartment for nonpayment of rent. Brian had used a special community fund to get her rent and security in a new apartment. The fund is hard to access and Brian had worked hard to get both the apartment and the money. The presentation focused on the client's unhappiness with the apartment and her demand for new furniture. The group members volunteered ideas about other available resources to meet her need. After the discussion had gone on for a while, the supervisor asked Brian how he felt about working with this client. Brian responded that she had a history of mental illness, was alienated from her family, and it was understandable that she was not satisfied. Linda agreed that it was understandable, but she felt irritated with the client and felt that at least a part of her would want to confront the client and point out her ingratitude. Another worker agreed, stating on the one hand you understand the clinical piece, but on the other, how can so many clients be ungrateful? The discussion on feeling put upon went on for several minutes as staff vented their frustrations. Linda summed up by saying, "We are all human and our feelings are understandable. Luckily we have knowledge of human behavior which helps us not react with our gut feeling."

In this example, Linda allows the "unmentionable" and in sanctioning the discussion is able to help her staff acknowledge feelings and move beyond them to a helping model.

In summary, group supervision offers both the supervisor and supervisees time-saving learning, and an opportunity to learn new skill sets. It offers the supervisor a new view of her workers, an opportunity to model good practice and a chance to uncover obstacles to learning. It helps the staff feel empowered to articulate difficult issues and feelings, and learn from each other.

Chapter 10

Difficult Conversations

Few people in the helping professions feel comfortable instigating conversations that are likely to cause anger or distress to clients or supervisees. When the issue is illegal or unethical behavior, the necessity for the conversation overrides any discomfort the supervisor or worker might feel. However, most problematic issues are not so clear-cut. Wanting to be sensitive to individual needs and the right to freedom of expression, needing to be liked and fearing the relationship will be irrevocably damaged if the subject is broached, supervisors and workers are liable to let problematic issues pass—hoping that they will resolve themselves even as they border on the inappropriate or potentially harmful.

A common supervisory error is to avoid difficult conversations as long as possible, and then let loose when a "last straw" event occurs. Unprepared and out of control, the supervisor thrashes about for examples of past behavior she did not mention before. Attacked and threatened, the worker responds with anger or mute dismay. The ill will generated from such unsatisfactory encounters is not easily undone. A common worker error is to observe potentially destructive situations (such as the possibility of alcoholism or an abusive family member) without discussing them with the client or supervisor.

Here, as in other chapters throughout this text, the issues faced by supervisor and worker are different, but there is a parallel process in resolving them. Unlike other chapters in this book, we lead with a discussion of the issue as it evolves in supervision, and follow with a translation of the principles to practice situations.

Gerontological Supervision
© 2008 by The Haworth Press, Taylor & Francis Group. All rights reserved.
doi:10.1300/5153_10

IN SUPERVISION

Typical scenarios: A competent and loving home care worker is frequently late to her client's home but the supervisor knows that she is a single mother with a disabled child whom she must get ready for school. A new and promising case manager makes home visits dressed in provocative halters and low-riding jeans, but after all she is only twenty-two and that is how her contemporaries dress. The nursing assistant who performs her tasks with skill and compassion habitually accompanies her actions with the quotation of biblical verses and reassurance of the wonders of heaven; religious belief that is the source of her commitment to a difficult job. A case manager who has done first-rate work in the past is going through a divorce, has taken many sick days, and when she is in the office seems to be preoccupied and uninvolved.

Then the home care worker is late one morning and the client burns herself trying to make coffee. The young case manager threatens to quit after the "groping" of a new male client. The nursing assistant is indignant when a resident's daughter tells her to stop "proselytizing." The inattentive case manager suddenly leaves the job and her caseload is found to be neglected. The supervisor who has recognized, but not addressed, the problem must now do so under pressure and on the defensive—for if she knew of the problem before, why did she let the situation continue?

Some problems may result from an employee's lack of clear expectations of what is and what is not considered appropriate workplace behavior. Job descriptions, orientation publications, and in-service discussions that include attendance requirements, dress codes, and possible conversational pitfalls offer the worker some direction and provide the supervisor with requirements she can refer back to.

Workers inevitably bring personal issues to the workplace; illness, family emergencies, and financial concerns that get in the way of their job performance. Although employee assistance programs are not always available in small health care or social service settings, linkages can be created to community agencies so that workers can be referred in times of need.

Even though it is possible to anticipate some situations and plan for them, there will always be some difficult conversations that cannot be avoided. While there is no script available, the following steps will get you on your way.

1. *Have you established that the problematic behaviors are habitual and potentially harmful through repeated observation and confidential consultation with colleagues?*

Everyone has "off" days. Determining that the behavior is a pattern—and identifying specific instances of when it occurs is the first step. Supervisors inevitably have personal biases—some of which may influence how they perceive the behaviors of those they supervise. Confidentially checking one's perceptions with colleagues and documenting when and how the problem affects services to clients is essential before deciding to raise the issue with a worker.

2. *When and how can the issue best be addressed?*

Think through the advantages and disadvantages of the many venues available. Written and oral communications, individual and group meetings, as part of a regular supervisory meeting or as a "stand-alone" communication are all options. If the issue is one that comes under the general rubric of "professional use of self" and is shared by others in the agency, it might best be addressed in a staff meeting or training session. Addressing the subject (dress codes, and boundaries between personal and on-the-job behaviors) with a group rather than an individual worker forestalls defensiveness. Co-workers may also yield insights and compromises that the supervisor might not have thought of independently.

3. *If the issue is clearly an individual one, when is the best time to bring it up?*

Once you have established that the issue is an individual pattern that adversely affects service delivery and must be addressed, it is necessary to plan a time and place to discuss it. If an evaluation conference is coming up, it provides a perfect opportunity. The worker who has first heard of her strengths is better able to hear areas that need improvement and a timetable for monitoring these efforts is an expected outcome. If an evaluation conference is not in the offing, the supervisor can raise the issue during a regularly scheduled conference or plan a separate meeting. In either case, it is a good idea to allow more time than you may need.

4. *Remember: It is the behavior, not the person, that is the problem.*

Being called to task by one's supervisor is a powerful blow to the self-esteem, recalling similar occasions by authority figures in the past. Presenting the problem as one correctable flaw in an otherwise satisfactory (perhaps superior) performance goes a long way toward supporting the worker's sense of competence even as she hears of her difficulties.

5. *State the problem simply and specifically; sit calmly and wait for the response.*

Rather than speak generally of the problem of "lateness," be prepared with concrete examples: dates, minutes or hours lost, and their consequences. There is no reason to present the problem apologetically or preface it with what you imagine might be your worker's responses. "I know you have a disabled child at home and that you have no help in the morning, but, really it is important that . . ." displays your discomfort with the conversation. It also assumes that you understand the worker's point of view. Which you don't. Yet.

6. *Actively listen to the worker's response. Explore what you do not understand.*

Even though it might be difficult, do not interrupt when you feel that your position is misstated or you are being unfairly accused. (This will shift the focus from the problem to the supervisory relationship.)

7. *Make sure you understand the worker's point of view through summing up what you thought you heard.*

Help the worker articulate her point of view. "What I hear you saying is that since you sometimes stay overtime in the evenings, you figured it was okay to come late in the morning? Did I get it right?" At this point the worker may add new information. Keep summing up until you both are clear on the problem and the worker's point of view.

8. *Ask the worker how she thinks the problem can best be resolved.*

As you see yourself as a helping professional, you probably have ideas as to how the worker can be best helped. The distracted case manager going through a divorce might benefit from therapy. The burdened home attendant might benefit from parenting classes. Gratuitous observations do more harm than good. Unless the worker has asked for your opinion, there is no reason to invade the worker's personal space and blur the professional boundary.

9. *Collaborate with the worker on a remedial plan with specific goals and a time frame for achieving them. Reach an agreement, how it will be monitored, and when you will meet again to review.*

The best plan of action starts with the worker's ideas. If these are vague ("I'll try to do better") insist on a specific, measurable course of action. If the worker is committed to change but unable to come up with a plan, you can then make suggestions. The case manager who dresses inappropriately may say that she is poor from paying off student loans and cannot afford "a whole new wardrobe." A few simple blouses that she can put on over her customary attire "like a uniform" for home visits may be all that is needed. (When the worker responds to your suggestion "yes, but," return to Steps 6 and 7. You are not yet in agreement.)

10. *Immediately after the meeting, make a written record of the conversation, be sure to include how it was resolved and next steps.*

Emotions run high in difficult conversations. Supervisors and workers may emerge with very different impressions of what took place. So it is important to get your version down as completely and clearly as you can. This record may be solely for your own files—a guide to return to if you are called to recollect what happened. The record may be shared with the worker or, if required by the agency, a part of the employee file.

Following the steps outlined does not guarantee a successful outcome. The worker might still react with anger or distress. As with other interventions, all that the supervisor can control is the process. If the process has been followed, most workers will feel supported and valued, even as they learn of behaviors they must change. For the few workers who do not, Step 10—written documentation in the employee file—will assure all who review the situation that the worker has received a fair hearing and opportunity to improve.

IN PRACTICE

Holding difficult conversations is also a problem for workers. Not wanting to upset the elder or arouse anger on the part of their family members, perhaps even afraid that contact with their agencies will be terminated, or that they will be liable for professional censure, they may keep delaying the conversation in the hope that an opportune moment will arise.

Typical scenarios: A participant of the Alzheimer's Day Program likes to be touched by the staff but winces and shrinks back when her son-in-law comes to take her home. The visually impaired home care client has cigarette butts mixed in with the coins on her bureau.

Like supervisors, workers may make observations, but let situations slide until a crisis forces them to confront them. The Alzheimer's client shows up with bruises and an examination reveals abuse. The home care client sets off a small fire in her room. When the client is injured as a result of a recognized but unaddressed situation, it is an unending source of remorse to the worker.

Other situations may not be as obviously harmful, but sensitive nevertheless. Inappropriate sexual advances, family conflicts over end-of-life care, and expression or acting out of racist attitudes are issues that need to be addressed with care.

While the steps outlined previously in this chapter are generally applicable, modifications are necessary. Unlike workers, clients may not be cognitively able to follow the process. Family members may be physically threatening.

The supervisor has a crucial role in helping her workers conduct difficult conversations with clients and family members. A common situation is the community elder who refuses needed care—steadfastly denying that anything is wrong. The more the worker points out the reasons for and benefits of additional services, the more the elder is forced to defend his position. An unproductive tug-of-war then ensues.

Richard, a case manager, complained to his supervisor that Mr. W. would not "listen to reason" and insisted that he was managing just fine when it was evident that he could not maintain the most basic level of safety and nutrition without assistance. The supervisor asked what Mr. W. feared would happen if he let someone in to help. Richard realized that he had been so intent in pointing out the positives of help that he had not thought to explore. When Richard did so, he learned that Mr. W.'s primary concern was how he could afford to pay. Information on his eligibility for publicly funded help went a long way toward helping him accept an attendant.

Workers, like supervisors, bring their own personal biases to practice. They may believe that older people should not drink at all, or misperceive the reactions of a demented elder. Checking their perceptions over time and with others who have contact with the client and family is essential.

Any approach should be discussed in supervision before bringing it to the client or family. The first issue to be considered is to whom the observation is to be communicated. (Does the client have the ability to participate in a discussion? If not, who else in the client's informal network of family and friends can be involved?) Next is, how should the situation be presented? The supervisor might want to accompany the worker (or provide security) if a threatening response—as in the case of suspected elder abuse—is anticipated.

Older people are aware of their vulnerability to abuse. Sometimes elders' fears lead them to see abuse where there is none. Just as often, there is real abuse and elders feel too intimidated or dependent upon the abuser to voice their situation. Either way, the steps to uncovering the real situation and intervening appropriately require many difficult conversations.

Abuse can be physical (striking or rough handling), verbal (humiliating or infantilizing an elder), withholding care, sexual, or theft of property. There are obvious signs of abuse. Evidence of physical abuse includes reports by the elder, bruises, burns, lacerations, or fractures. Verbal abuse could be evidenced by elder reporting, anxiety around the caretaker, overdependence on visitors, concerns of neighbors, or other caregivers. Malnutrition, dehydration, weight loss or gain, skin breakdown, signs of over or under use of medications may be evidence of withholding treatment. Anxiety, injury to genitals, or excessive interest in sex may indicate sexual abuse. Loss of valuables, articles of sentimental value, or money may be evidence of theft.

The dilemma for the care manager is that all of these signs may indicate symptoms of normal physical deterioration and/or cognitive loss. Thus, there is the need for difficult conversations with the elder, with the caregiver, and/or with the family member. With the elder, the conversation is to encourage as many specific details as possible about an incident.

Lara, case manager for a home care agency, investigated a report of physical abuse reported by an anxious daughter. She asked Mrs. K. about her bath the day before. Mrs. K. told her that she had been watching her favorite soap opera when the attendant told her she needed to take a bath immediately. When Mrs. K. refused, the attendant turned off the television, wheeled her to the bath, and began to undress her. Mrs. K. fought back and when she was held down began screaming. A neighbor knocked on the door and then called Mrs. K.'s daughter.

Lara then spoke to the home attendant who was clearly frightened and defensive. In recounting what happened, she said that Mrs. K. was incontinent and needed changing in addition to a bath. She had already waited half an hour and was fearful that there would be another skin breakdown. Mrs. K.'s daughter had already threatened to fire her when there was a reddened area on her mother's buttock.

Lara removed the attendant from Mrs. K.'s home. She also recommended in-service training and careful monitoring. While the attendant had used poor judgment, she was not a volatile or random abuser. Lara then called Mrs. K.'s daughter and discussed the need for them to work together in monitoring her mother's care.

Neil, social worker in a nursing facility, followed up on a family complaint that their very confused mother had suddenly started using explicitly sexual language. He asked the family to give him specifics about her words and contents. He also asked the staff who said that sexual offers often accompanied personal care and bathing. Knowing the resident's background, Neil concluded that the behavior was more than a breakdown of inhibitions. He focused in on a friendly male visitor who had started visiting this resident a few months ago. In asking about the context of their conversation, it became clear that the visitor misconstrued the resident's interest in him as an interest in his sexual life. He had answered her inquiries in great detail.

Neil removed this volunteer and worked with the volunteer director to address difficult topics in training. He also successfully advocated for supervision of new volunteers who would visit confused residents. He advised the resident's family and hands-on staff to redirect her comments. The sexual content of the resident's conversation disappeared in a short time.

Jenna, Director of an Adult Day Care Center, followed up on a family member's complaint and found that the supervisory structure of her program was in disarray. A daughter reported that her mother had lost $100 the last time she attended the program. The daughter was angry with the program supervisor who had told them that her mother should not carry that much money. The nursing assistant was also angry with the supervisor who had asked her if the member had a purse with her when the assistant took her to the bathroom. Jenna gave the member $100 in reimbursement. Recognizing that the supervisor bypassed the member, alienated the family, and alienated the nursing assistant, she met alone with her to talk about the need to explore a problem, ask details, and investigate before reacting with defensiveness and accusation. Jenna soon discovered that the supervisor who seemed very confident often felt unsure of how to respond to conflict. The supervisor was relieved to learn that she did not have to handle everything alone and could turn to the Director when things "got out of hand." Bimonthly supervisory sessions were also scheduled. (The daughter sent a check when she found the "missing" money in her mother's jewelry box.)

This example looks at two aspects of our culture that often get in the way of good practice. It may not be wise in the world we live in to carry cash, but a defensive "blame the victim" response is not going to solve any problems. Similarly, the assumption that the underprivileged, nonprofessional worker is a thief, promotes stereotypical, prejudiced thinking. Jenna had a significant amount of work to do with this supervisor.

Substance abuse is likely to involve many difficult conversations. It may involve lifelong alcoholism or a drinking problem that manifested itself in late life. Alcoholism may mask untreated psychiatric problems. More commonly in the elderly, substance abuse is an inability to realize the impact of alcohol on an aging mind and body. Substance abuse may also involve an overreliance on prescription drugs.

An older client with lifelong substance abuse problems will come into a care system with a history and related diagnoses. The treatment plan will need to take the history into account. Successful interventions (AA for example) should be continued as part of a care plan. Monitoring of lab work and the disease process will indicate any emerging problems. The case manager will need to have an open discussion about substance abuse history with the client and family. He will reinforce the need to follow the care plan and the consequences of deviating from it. A psychiatric assessment of the client is an important part of the care plan. Alcohol is often the treatment of choice for depression and alcohol abuse is common among the mentally ill. Treatment of the underlying psychiatric issue can make an enormous difference in the well-being of a previously undiagnosed elder.

Moderate social drinkers need to understand the impact of alcohol on the aging body and mind. Sometimes simple education is a quick and easy answer. Elders may decide to switch from martinis to sherry when they are educated on the impact of hard liquor on their systems.

Elders with physical impairments need little discussion to recognize that a fall could land them in a wheelchair. Elders with cognitive impairment make education harder and sometimes need more focused intervention.

The nurse manager alerted Helen, the home care social worker, to a problem that often occurred on the night shift. Mr. B., an eighty-four-year-old with dementia, and in the early stages of Parkinson's disease, was often asleep when the attendant arrived, a half-filled water sized glass of vodka by his side. Helen spoke with Mr. B. who assured her he had not had a drink in ten years. She spoke with his son who said that his parents had cocktails before dinner every night, but had never been abusers. He was also concerned, as his father did not remember what he ate or drank. Anne continued her inquiry with Mr. B.'s physician who said that the patient's cognitive state impaired his judgment about alcohol use. She then spoke directly to Mr. B. explaining that his memory was not as good as it used to be and that his physician thought alcohol was hurting him. She asked him what he thought was a solution. The client said he always followed his doctor's advice. His son removed the alcohol. His home care worker added a "Virgin" Mary to his dinner menu. His son offered a predinner drink when they went out to dinner.

Difficult conversations often become easier when everyone, including the impaired elder, is involved in the conversation, has the opportunity to express his or her point of view, and can "own" a plan. An impaired person, like Mr. B., will typically ask for a drink the next day, but can be reminded each time of his doctor's advice. An elder who reports abuse must be taken seriously each and every time. However, the investigation should be objective, thorough, and not impacted by previous inaccurate reports. The case manager who identifies the difficult issues early and intervenes quickly will find these "difficult" conversations will quickly become routine.

Part IV:
Supervising Interns

Chapter 11

Assignment Selection

Agencies take on the education of interns for many reasons: to increase services to clients, to add to agency prestige through collaboration with a professional school, and to develop the skills of their workers—skills that are also useful in staff supervision.

In educational supervision, the agency is a laboratory in which theories learned at school are put to the test—and additional knowledge and skills are imparted. The excitement in gerontological education is that something new is uncovered all the time, with new theories and practice approaches springing up from unexpected sources. Highly experienced supervisors *haven't* seen it all before.

ASSIGNMENT SELECTION

The first question that the school asks of the supervisor and the supervisor needs to decide is: What tasks are appropriate for assignment to an intern? Coming up with a caseload that is "real life" yet not overwhelming, which contains sufficient learning opportunities without

Gerontological Supervision
© 2008 by The Haworth Press, Taylor & Francis Group. All rights reserved.
doi:10.1300/5153_11

posing risk to client or intern, and that is either outside the concerns of reimbursement sources or is accepted by them (with the obligatory "sign off" of an accredited professional) is challenging. Combined with the problem of finding time within one's own schedule and patience within oneself to supervise a beginner for whom no knowledge can be assumed deters many would-be educational supervisors from an enriching experience.

THE SUPERVISOR'S CHALLENGE

Every agency administrator and supervisor can think of a "wish list"—nonreimbursable services that would benefit the population if resources could only be found. The presence of an intern can allow many of these wishes to come true. A nursing intern in a home care setting may institute a series of meetings for family members—helping them to better understand their elder's medical problems and daily care needs. A social work intern in a nursing home can run a group of community spouses. A research study of patients discharged from a hospital with home care may measure the effectiveness of home-based services. These and other interventions often happen only because of the intern's presence in an agency and, in many ways, change the course of gerontological practice.

Unfortunately, few agencies offer the long-term services of a professional worker to the elderly and their families. Of this small group, even fewer document their interventions. The intern experience with the elderly offers an arena for new ideas to be tested, and an opportunity to generate more advanced clinical thinking.

The supervisor in charge of practicum instruction (sometimes known as the field instructor or field educator) is accountable to her agency to provide the best possible service to the client group. At the same time, she is accountable to the school and to the intern to provide a valid learning experience. So in developing an assignment, she will consider the educational needs of the intern as well as the service needs of the agency. In addition, the supervisor can design an assignment which may challenge existing assumptions or augment the literature in gerontological practice.

Ideally, the assignment will expose the intern to a wide range of elderly clients, needs, and intervention modalities. This would include clients of various races, ethnicities, income levels, and ages, men and women, couples and families, in the community and in institutions, faced with developmental crises and situational crises. This varied population would be amenable to short- and long-term interventions either individually or in groups.

In reality, the extent of exposure is limited by the kind of population the agency serves, as well as the type of client the agency staff sees as needing help. Frail, very old widows who have difficulty in adapting to institutional living may predominate in nursing home referrals. Socially isolated elders may similarly predominate in the community. Group services are rare in community agencies where home visits are the norm. Service to families may be nonreimbursable and not offered on a routine basis either in the community or institution.

Moreover, agency service needs usually encompass a range of administrative tasks—such as compliance with government and board directives, recordings—beyond interaction with clients. The agency standards for performance relate to what the staff member accomplished for the client within a specified time. Educational expectations have a very different emphasis. There is still the demand to meet administrative requirements. However, satisfaction in an assignment relates to the process of the work and what the intern learns.

The initial task for the practicum instructor, then, is to assess agency and educational needs, and negotiate for assignments amenable to both parties.

A few questions to consider:

> What was the previous agency experience with interns?
> What assignments met the interns' learning needs and had meaning to the agency?
> What assignments did not work out? Why did they fail?
> What could have improved a particular assignment?
> What is not being done that an intern could initiate?
> If interns have been in a particular service for several years—is it still a good use of student time? Is the outcome productive?
> What information do I have about this intern, and how can I use it?

Answers to these questions are combined with thinking related to the particular needs of the arriving students:

> Could this nursing staff handle a beginner who has no experience with the elderly?
> Has anyone initiated a program in this service before?
> Has research ever been a part of this program?

BALANCING SERVICE NEEDS AND LEARNING OPPORTUNITIES

The student's educational plan will be determined by collaboration between the school and agency. Most schools expect that assignments will increase in number and complexity as the intern progresses through the practicum, and that the intern will have an opportunity to demonstrate his understanding of classroom work through practice with individuals in the field. Beyond that, it is up to the supervisor (field instructor or practicum instructor) to balance the service needs of clients with the learning needs of students. This is not always easy.

If the supervisor chooses cases based only on service needs (selecting those clients who are in greatest need of help) the intern may be ineffective and discouraged by professional expectations beyond his capacity. He may also end up with a caseload composed of similar clients facing similar situations (say, end-of-life issues) with little or no exposure to the range of concerns faced by ill and disabled older people and their families. If the supervisor chooses cases based only on learning needs (selecting cases because they are "interesting" or "not too difficult" or offer broad exposure to the field) the assignment will not reflect a real situation—and it is a real practice situation for which the interns are preparing. So it is most important to identify the learning opportunity within each service need.

The beginning intern will profit from a broad introduction to common clinical situations and the health care system to be found in situations such as these:

Mr. G., a sixty-five-year-old chronic alcoholic, is a new admission to a nursing home. He is scapegoated by other residents and staff. The service need is to help Mr. G. adapt to a new living arrangement, monitor his alcoholism, and develop an individualized assessment and case plan. The learning need is to understand alcoholism in the elderly, learn treatment interventions, and gain knowledge of group dynamics and the scapegoating process.

Mrs. L. is an eighty-year-old mildly confused woman whose daughters referred her to a community agency for help with placement. She wishes to maintain her own apartment and appears able to do this with appropriate supports. The service need is to develop a workable plan to maintain her safety and interpret her care needs to the family. The learning need is knowledge of the mentally frail, development of resources, and skill in work with the family unit.

A support group for older people with macular degeneration. The service need is to provide a forum for members to share their concerns and receive practical tips in dealing with their situations. The learning need is understanding the skills of group work and the psychosocial issues surrounding vision impairment.

Advanced cases can be more complex—featuring a number of issues and requiring a greater depth of psychosocial understanding and gerontological knowledge.

Mr. and Mrs. R., a couple in their eighties, were referred to a community agency. Mrs. R. is physically ill and confused. Mr. R. is attempting unsuccessfully to care for her, but is perpetually at war with the home care attendant who comes to help (and is now threatening to leave). There is no close family. The service need is to develop a care plan for Mrs. R., and help Mr. R. accept her needs and his own limitations as well as mediate between the couple and the direct care worker. The learning need is understanding and utilizing the underlying dynamics of the relationship along with mediating skills.

Mrs. Z., the seventy-year-old daughter of a nursing home patient spends the better part of her time on the unit, criticizing the medical care of her mother and frequently disrupting the floor staff by demanding changes in treatment. The service need is helping Mrs. Z. learn how to advocate for her mother in the setting and easing her relationship with the staff. The learning need is an assessment of the mother-daughter relationship and developing appropriate intervention strategies with family and staff.

Developing an outreach program to the community. The service need is making individuals and institutions aware of the agency's services and stimulating referrals. The learning need is enhancing organizational and communication skills.

It is rarely possible, or even desirable, to have a complete assignment developed by the time the intern arrives. Most often, assignments are developed within the first six weeks as the intern's interests and abilities surface during the preliminary educational assessment. Assignments are then developed with the following considerations in mind.

What does the intern need to know? When must he know it? Field education is primarily experiential. Interns are expected to meet face-to-face with a client—and to project a professional image—within the first weeks of field placement. However, they differ in how well they are prepared. Some may come directly from undergraduate school and have no comparable experience. Some may have several years of work experience in a related field and have returned to school to gain necessary credentials. Still others may have work experience in an unrelated field (such as sales) where interactional skills differ from those of the helping professions.

Evaluation criteria provided by the school indicate the minimal standards for acceptable practice; yet minimal criteria do not accurately reflect the differing abilities of a natural beginner or the struggle of a highly experienced returnee to move beyond preconceived notions. Gerontological education, like gerontological practice, is based on an individualized assessment.

The expectations for practice will depend on the intern's background, experience, intellectual ability, and understanding of the field. Initially, the supervisor uses the information from the school, as well as the intern's initial presentation, to begin the educational assessment. Of particular concern for the beginning assessment is how the individual learns best.

DIFFERENT TYPES OF LEARNERS AND THEIR BEGINNINGS WITH CLIENTS

The intuitive learner will be most comfortable getting "in there" with the client, and pulling out issues from the experience. The intellectual learner will need more theoretical knowledge before beginning. The practical learner will respond best to immediate, clear feedback, and can most benefit from role-play before the first encounter.

Mrs. K., an eighty-nine-year-old widow living alone with housekeeping assistance is referred to a community mental health center by her physician because she seems depressed and isolated. Each intern would begin with her somewhat differently.

Joan, a first-year intern with a background in journalism, is quick to involve herself at the agency and can hardly wait to meet her first client. Encouraged by the supervisor to go in and listen, she is comfortable asking Mrs. K. to talk about herself. She also makes many observations of Mrs. K. and her environment. In reviewing the process recording with her supervisor, Joan can look at Mrs. K.'s words and situation and understand her difficulty coping with changes in her life as her health declines.

Assigned to David who entered social work school after completing a degree in philosophy, Mrs. K. would wait a little longer for service. She would meet her worker after he learned enough about depression in the aged to assess the possibility of either a reactive or endogenous depression. Although David could not learn everything before the first meeting, he would be more comfortable knowing that physical illness, poor nutrition, and social isolation are all common causes of depression-like symptoms in the elderly. With Mrs. K., he will ask questions designed to identify symptoms of depression. Eliminating clinical symptoms, David will look for socioenvironmental factors as clues for work.

Margaret is a second-year intern with a teaching background. She knows that supervision will help her to understand and help Mrs. K. As Mrs. K., in a role-play situation, she begins to imagine how Mrs. K. might feel. As herself again, she notes her supervisor's responses and concerns as Mrs. K.

None of these categories is, of course, absolute. The intellectual learner gets his questions from experience. The intuitive learner must know enough about depression in the elderly to recognize symptoms. The practical learner uses a combination of experience and intellect. Thus, the supervisor who can assess how best the student learns will move the student more quickly down his educational path.

Chapter 12

The Supervisory Conference and Recording Requirements

THE SUPERVISORY CONFERENCE

The core tension in educational supervision, at least at the beginning, is often the supervisor's certainty that learning must come from the intern and the intern's equal certainty that the supervisor can and must tell him what to do. The social work perspective on supervision is, for most beginning interns, a learning experience unlike any they have known before. In the classroom, the instructor communicates information to the student who demonstrates learning through exams and papers. In the field, the worker is monitored to see that he performs his work in a timely, effective manner. Yet in educational supervision the intern is expected to record and reflect on his interactions with clients and staff—including his opinions and feelings. He may be puzzled or angered by the process. Why are answers being withheld when the supervisor obviously knows them?

This anxiety is compounded by the content to be taught. In most professions, the subject material is acknowledged as specialized and available only to those who have made a concentrated study of the area. It is possible to identify the moment when one has passed from not knowing to knowing how to conduct a cross-examination or fill a cavity. Clinical skills are different. Their acquisition is a subtle process of blending professional values, knowledge, and skills with the individual character of the practitioner. It is this that is referred to as the "professional use of self."

As learning is gradual, uneven, and evident in some areas before others, it is difficult for the student to realize when it occurs. What is

Gerontological Supervision
© 2008 by The Haworth Press, Taylor & Francis Group. All rights reserved.
doi:10.1300/5153_12

more, when close supervisory attention is paid to his personal reactions to clients, the intern may feel that his privacy is being invaded. Most important, he may feel that a judgment of his work is a judgment of his character.

With all of this in mind, the supervisor must be clear in explaining the purpose, content, and process of conferences. To tell a beginning intern that learning must come from him is useless and anxiety provoking. In the beginning, he may not even know what he should know or how to frame questions to get the answers he needs.

A description of clinical skills and how they can be learned in supervision will offer the student both intellectual content and assurance that the supervisor can help.

Beginning with a first-year intern, the supervisor explained that they would begin by engaging the client. She asked the intern how she thought that an elderly patient could be engaged. Isolated in a nursing home, they agreed that the patient might be happy to see anyone. On the other hand, the supervisor noted the physical impairments common to the elderly which can make communication difficult. She suggested talking clearly, repeating, and changing phrasing to ensure that the client understands.

In the preceding example, the supervisor prefaces the discussion with identification of the skill to be learned: engagement. She then draws on the intern's experience and common sense to develop professional skill. Finally, she offers professional knowledge and gerontological expertise to help the intern learn.

The supervisor must also be sensitive to the intern's reactions to first experiences in the field. Work with the aging often awakens troubling feelings in the intern. Nevertheless, supervision is not therapy, and time spent on personal issues must be designated as such.

The supervisor noted that Jane's eyes filled with tears as she recounted her interview with Mrs. Y. who she said reminded her of her late grandmother. The supervisor noted that Jane's reactions to clients were often personal and wondered if that had to do with the fact that they were elderly. Jane said it did, and talked at length about how respect for the old was insisted upon in her family. Often it was hard for her to make demands on clients. She was aware, in fact, that she would sometimes not raise issues if she thought her client would get angry. She mentioned that this was not the case with Mrs. Y., because her grandmother never was angry with her. The supervisor suggested they take a five-minute break from the work. She said she would like to know more about Jane's grandmother and other people in her family if she would like to tell her.

The supervisor was careful to preface this time-out discussion with an explanation that personal experiences and feelings often get in the way of the work. Identifying differences between one's own family and the client population is necessary. Thus, Jane heard that her whole life was not up for discussion; her feelings about elders would only be examined as they affected her practice.

THE CONFERENCE AGENDA

Supervisory and intern agendas guarantee that the conference will cover all that needs to be discussed in a timely and focused manner. The intern's agenda—submitted in advance—is a useful tool for the supervisor in understanding what the intern sees as his learning need and how he formulates areas of interest and concern. In the beginning, agenda items are usually practical (how to get a food stamp application) or globally complex (do the K.s need marriage counseling and how should I begin?).

The supervisor uses the agenda items as a point of departure to respond to the intern's worries, discover what information is needed, and to teach conceptual thinking. In the case of food stamps, it may be a matter of directing the intern to a resource library to develop knowledge of all the entitlements available to the population. In the case of marital counseling, the supervisor can explore the student's understanding of the clients' problems and suggest items for the next conference. "Think about what aspects of couple's counseling might be useful or unclear to you and we will focus on them next week." The intern is then encouraged to think of practice in a more specific way.

By the end of the first semester, the intern should be submitting agendas with specific queries that can be used as the foundation of experiential exercises.

How do I engage Mrs. M.'s son to plan with Mrs. M. when he responds "ask my sister."

How do I encourage Mrs. M.'s daughter to include her brother and share her caregiving role?

The supervisor's agenda uses the intern's agenda as a point of departure but moves beyond it to incorporate knowledge and skills that are not only relevant to the case at hand but are applicable to the population in general. In Mrs. M.'s case described previously, this would involve knowledge of common dynamics of the aging family and intervention skills.

RECORDING

Interns often prefer to talk about their work rather than writing about it. While the supervisor's immediate input is often necessary for a timely intervention, habitual reliance on "talking about" robs the conference of much of its teaching potential.

Audio and video tape, summary recording, and process recording—used singly or in combination—are all appropriate methods of capturing the intern's work with clients.

Taping is especially useful in developing self-awareness. The intern can observe himself and the client at a distance—free of the anxiety of the interview situation. It can also be useful to the supervisor, revealing small but significant nonverbal and verbal interactions that might not be captured in written form. Drawbacks to the use of tape are financial (they may be costly), practical (they take more time to review), and legal (they require releases from clients). Moreover, they are inappropriate for many elders and settings.

Summary Recordings are useful for teaching interns how to conceptualize and condense their observations—skills that are necessary for chart notes and other forms of recording required by agencies and funders. Summary recordings can also keep supervisors apprised of developments in cases that, for lack of time, cannot be process recorded each week.

Process Recordings are extensively used in the education of social work interns. The process recording can be a narrative of the interview.

"Mr. P. was thirty minutes late for the appointment. He began with a long diatribe against the 'access a ride' program and I urged him to calm down."

Or it can be in a script-like format.

MR. P: I can't believe how incompetent those people are. They were not only late, they sent an inexperienced driver who had no idea how to handle my wheelchair.

ME: I'm sure they did the best they could. You should really try to relax.

Process recording can be used differentially, depending on the intern's learning needs. A student needing to work on empathizing with the client will frequently benefit from line by line review with a focus on recreating the experience.

SUPERVISOR: How did you feel when he told you about his experience with access a ride? What did he look like then? How would you feel in his place? What would you want to hear from the person to whom you told your story?

In the case of a more empathic student (frequently an intuitive learner) who was able to respond to Mr. P.'s distress, the teaching point might be to move beyond the individual situation to generalize—what did this experience reveal about Mr. P.'s strengths and areas of difficulty or about areas in the service system that need to be addressed?

It is not helpful to give back recording with comments before supervision. The intern may try to explain away his problems, feel like a failure, or not develop his own ideas. Even positive comments are less than helpful because the intern often does not know why an intervention was good or how he can repeat it. However, reviewing a process recording with comments after supervision can augment or reinforce some of the discussion.

Interns often fear that they will not remember exactly what happened; yet verbatim replication is not the purpose of the process recording. Rather, the intern reproduces what he recalls as important even if he does not recognize or respond to its significance while the interview is taking place. The supervisor is then able to bring the issue into awareness.

In Jim's recording, he kept telling Mrs. W. all the services the agency could offer while Mrs. W. responded by talking about how well-off she was compared with other older people. Jim's accurate rendering (if not understanding) of the communication problem opened the door to a productive supervisory discussion.

Chapter 13

Group Supervision, Evaluation

GROUP SUPERVISION

When there are several interns placed at an agency, group supervision is a useful adjunct to individual supervision. It need not necessarily take more time. Shaving some time off individual supervisory conferences and using it for weekly or biweekly group sessions can be very effective.

GETTING STARTED

Group meetings can be structured in many ways to serve many ends. At the beginning of the internship, it can be a vehicle for orientation to the agency and preparation for initial work with clients. Lectures on different aspects of the agency's work and distribution of written materials are the easiest ways to do this. Unfortunately, these methods can grow boring and interns retain little. Participatory exercises ensure enthusiasm and hasten the formation of group cohesiveness.

Interns may be asked to keep logs during the first week or two in the agency. In them, they can record all their impressions and questions and share them with the group. They may be sent on teams with a list of questions to explore the community or the long-term care facility in which they are placed. When they return they will have information to contribute; the ways in which they do this help the supervisor ascertain their observational abilities and concerns. Interns may also participate in simulation exercises in which they must accomplish simple tasks wearing blindfolds, wax in their ears, or manipulate a

Gerontological Supervision
doi:10.1300/5153_13

wheelchair. Many find such experiences helpful in beginning to empathize with ill and disabled clients, whose worldview is so different from their own.

The supervisor might also experiment with an exercise on listening and responding to typical responses of elderly clients at first meetings with their assigned intern. One intern can be asked to play the client, another his worker. Then roles can be switched. A third intern can be a recorder, noting verbal and nonverbal aspects of the interaction. This exercise develops empathy while calling on the students' dramatic abilities and fostering camaraderie, this exercise is useful in developing empathy for clients while revealing areas in which they have difficulty.

When the interns are well into the work (usually after the first month), it is possible to shift to a practice conference format. This method can be related to a specific issue or focus on the practice of one intern each week. An issue-related group session will require brief presentations by each intern around one problem—such as communication with medical personnel. A group session devoted to the work of one intern will emphasize the importance of collaborative thinking on a work in progress rather than a judgment of performance. It will also provide interns with experience making professional presentations.

The supervisor fosters group discussion and mutual aid—underscoring general practice principles to be drawn from individual situations.

A group meeting for social work interns, early in the semester focused on how to obtain and use medical information. The supervisor offered and encouraged the interns to share their feelings about the physicians. She acknowledged that dismissive responses were not uncommon. Use of role-play helped the interns identify some reasons why physicians may respond the way they do. Interns were then able to identify points of common interest and work on how to present their questions and concerns effectively. Each had an opportunity to role-play the social worker and get feedback from others. The supervisor helped them identify skills needed to engage different professionals, and how to focus the conversation to foster information sharing. Since several interns worked with doctors who had been trained in other countries, she took the opportunity to comment on sociocultural differences as well as differences in professional education.

At a later meeting, one intern presented the case of Mrs. L., a mildly confused eighty-five-year-old woman who lived independently with a home health aide. Mrs. L.'s daughter—who had contracted with the agency—was concerned about her mother's gradual decline and wanted to discuss application to a long-term facility. The intern was upset that the daughter wanted to "ship" her mother to a home—a view initially shared by all the other interns. Advocating Mrs. L.'s right to "self-determination," they posed the problem as to whether they owed their allegiance to the client or her daughter. Role-play helped the interns understand the daughter's viewpoint. The supervisor's input on family systems theory—and the interdependence of family members throughout the life span—removed the case from an "either-or" situation to a consideration of how the intern could help mediate different perspectives on the situation. Emphasis on understanding client problems but not feeling the need to solve them was reinforced in the group.

Group supervision also provides interns with an experiential learning situation in developing group skills. As the intern sees himself and his peers act out group dynamics in a real-life situation, he also sees the supervisor modeling the group leader he will become.

GROUP PROJECTS

By midyear, it is useful to spend at least half of group supervision on a group project. The project provides students with a rewarding hands-on experience in practice research or organizational change. They learn to work together in making a lasting contribution to the agency or to the field. In the process, they discover the rewards and frustrations of such efforts.

The genesis of a project can come from many sources and fan out in many directions. Following is a list of some of the projects that our student units have accomplished as examples of what might be done.

Day-Care Expansion Project: providing a needs assessment of the community

Resident Council Project: analyzing the bylaws of the council, interviewing staff and residents, tracking one complaint through the council system

Discharge from Subacute Care: follow-up study of elders in the community who had been discharged from the rehabilitation unit of a hospital within the past year

Loss and Bereavement: an in-depth study of how various disciplines within a nursing home function when a resident dies

Interns often respond to the idea of a project hesitantly and fearfully. They may see little relevance to their clinical concerns. It sounds very hard and feels like a lot of extra work. However, a group project provides an opportunity for creativity and initiative that is not available in any other assignment. Although the supervisor is crucial in providing guidance and mediating disagreements, the group is responsible for task accomplishment. Students soon understand that the project will be as in-depth as they decide. They learn to use time productively and effectively.

As the supervisor helps the group break down the project into manageable pieces, she models the skill of partialization. As students develop tools to gather information and implement ideas, they also begin to identify individual interests and strengths. The supervisor soon sees areas of strength in some students that were not apparent in the individual work.

The interplay among group members becomes more dynamic as time goes on and the students live the group experience. The supervisor remains available, but is able to stand back and let the group develop on its own. Among the areas that the interns might learn about through the project are: clinical interventions, organizational theory, research methodologies, group process, and negotiating systems. In addition to the interns learning many skills, the group project may lead to longlasting organizational change.

EVALUATION

Note: The following section is based on a social work model that prevails in most graduate school programs. While we recognize that other health disciplines have different criteria and evaluation methods, the general principles may still apply.

An Ongoing Process

Evaluation of an intern, as evaluation of a worker, is an ongoing process. The supervisor is responsible for keeping the intern apprised of his progress so that there should be no surprises at either the mid-term or end-of-semester evaluation. Evaluation of an intern, as evaluation of a worker, is also a shared process. Mutuality is a difficult concept for many interns to understand. They often do not have the ability to judge their own work—and may only know what felt right or what went wrong. Nevertheless, with time and great individual variation, they become better able to identify practice skills and problems as related to the professional criteria by which they are evaluated.

Mid-Semester Evaluation

A written assessment early in the semester helps the supervisor clarify her thinking. It also gives the intern a written document to refer to when, because of anxiety or inexperience, she may not fully grasp the points cited in the oral evaluation. The mid-semester evaluation is typically held six weeks into the semester. While there has not yet been time enough to get a full picture of the intern's strengths and difficulties, an initial judgment can still be made. Most importantly, it allows the intern time before the end of the semester to work on problems that have been identified.

Six-Week Educational Assessment and Plan

Ellen Johnson, Clinical Practice

Second Year. November, 2006

Ms. Johnson came to the Hatfield Nursing Home with an interest in aging and a strong motivation to learn social work skills. Her first-year placement was with troubled adolescents and she had prior experience in a hospital. Ms. Johnson is dedicated and committed, easily involving herself in the agency and with the population, and quickly developed knowledge of policies and procedures. She is empathic in approach and communicates well. However, she needs more clarity about her role as a helping professional. She is quick to offer solutions before fully understanding the problem, and needs to concentrate during this semester on developing skills in exploring and reaching underlying feelings. Her capacity to assess environmental obstacles and strengths is well developed. In strengthening assessment skills, the focus will be on intrapsychic obstacles. Ms. Johnson is strong in identifying, and engaging services and resources. Although responsive in supervision, she is hesitant to offer her own opinions and ideas. Goals for the semester include: (1) developing her ability to explore client thoughts and feelings, (2) making more psychodynamic assessments, (3) staying with painful feelings of clients, and (4) taking more risks in the learning process. Ms Johnson's assignment consists of four long-term cases and one group (a Reminiscence Group on a skilled nursing unit). She will soon be assigned to telephone inquiry duty in the Intake Department to develop familiarity and ability with short-term assessment and intervention. Ms. Johnson has read and agreed with this evaluation and plan.

The mutual assessment process that leads to the six-week educational assessment and plan—with its bird's-eye view of the intern as a learner and practitioner—is a useful point of departure for discussion with the practicum advisor assigned by the school.

End-of-Semester Evaluation

As the semester draws to a close, the supervisor is charged with providing the school with a written critique of the intern's practice. Having gone through the process of evaluation with the student during the mid-semester oral evaluation, it is generally easy to begin a discussion of practice. However, the demand to provide a detailed account to the school is often anxiety producing to both supervisor and intern. No matter how much verbal feedback has been offered, the written evaluation represents a definitive representation of the intern's performance at a time when he is expected to have reached specific performance criteria as established by the school.

For the supervisor, particularly a beginning supervisor preparing the written evaluation often arouses latent feelings of inadequacy and insecurity. "Have I taught enough?" "Was I clear?" "Was I available enough" "Should I have done more?" Similarly, the intern may experience an anxious regression back to early school days when a teacher's approval of him was all-important. The wish to do well may thus supplant the ability of both supervisor and intern to assess the work and level of development. What is more, an intern who has returned to school after independent employment may have difficulty with the new role as a learner and become defensive or dismissive of the evaluation process.

The supervisor will first need to handle her own anxiety. Focusing on the importance of her professional role will allow her to be more objective in her responses. Similarly, the supervisor helps alleviate the intern's anxiety by structuring the evaluation process. She begins by providing specific steps to prepare for the evaluation conference.

Prior to the evaluation conference, the intern is asked to read the performance criteria for the semester and review all her recordings and case notes as well as her own recollection of significant developments in all her assignments. The supervisor, of course, does the same. The purpose of this review is twofold: to assess skills development in particular situations and over time.

As a result of this review, both supervisor and intern enter the conference prepared to discuss specific examples of the work that illustrate practice skills, growth in ability, or areas needing further development. It is best for the intern to go first with the supervisor hearing him out, demonstrating that evaluation is a mutual process. If the supervisor has already made up her mind, it will be evident to the intern. At the same time, the supervisor is a professional with professional standards to uphold. While the intern is entitled to a fair hearing—which often sheds light on areas that were previously unclear to the supervisor—the supervisor cannot let the intern control the process or dictate what should be included in the written evaluation.

How can the supervisor hear out the intern when she has already made a professional assessment? She can carefully and thoroughly explore the intern's comments and assessment of the work. Often the intern's thinking does not differ much from the supervisor's assessment, but needs to be conceptualized and identified as an issue for work.

Sally's supervisor asked her how she saw herself developing in group work. Sally said that she "loved" groups and felt her contracting and exploring was good. The supervisor asked what helped her. Sally talked about the receptivity of the members of the senior planning group and how much she liked them. The supervisor asked what was hard for her. Sally talked about difficulty dealing with other staff over scheduling and a few seniors who responded with anger when she suggested that they become more active. They agreed that Sally found negative reactions hard to understand or deal with and agreed on it as an area for future work.

Despite the demand for review of the work and self-analysis, interns may come to the evaluation conference unprepared or with vague, unfocussed self-observations: "I know I have a lot to learn" or "I finally think I know what I'm supposed to be doing." If the supervisor believes that the student is not taking responsibility, she can refuse to proceed with the conference and reschedule at a time when the intern is prepared to produce his own ideas.

The actual writing of the evaluation is the supervisor's job. Demands on the intern to do more than review and discuss his performance are inappropriate and unethical. The written evaluation is most effective when it looks at progress over time.

> Elaine's discomfort with the setting and the population was evident in her beginning practice. She viewed the client group stereotypically making assumptions about "old people's" needs and wants. Her attempts to stay with the clients' feelings and explore their concerns came across as insensitive and challenging rather than helpful. As Elaine became more familiar with the agency and responded to supervision, she began to see the population as individuals with particular problems and concerns. The group assignment was particularly useful to her in developing a sense of what a social worker does to help. Her strengths emerged in the group. As she experienced members responding when she "asked rather than told," she began to relax, and transferred skills developed in the group to practice with individuals.

Another intern's practice may be best understood in the context of patterns.

> Robert is not fully comfortable in the social work role. He has difficulty presenting himself as a professional and responds to clients more as a friendly visitor. This situation makes his interventions uneven. Good engagement skills are evident in his work; however, Robert moves away from exploring issues that are painful or conflicted. His ongoing work follows the same pattern of uneven interventions. Although he makes accurate assessments of his clients' needs and empathizes with their difficulties, he stops short of translating his knowledge into a plan of intervention.

When Problems Arise

There are many reasons why practitioners decide to supervise interns. It is gratifying to provide an atmosphere for learning, to teach skills, and to share one's practice wisdom. Assuming a nurturing supportive role with clients comes naturally to the clinician who works with ill and disabled elders and this role is easily translated to the supervisory experience. At the same time, practicum instruction is often the first time that the practitioner serves in an administrative role, occupying a position of sanctioned authority over others. The conflict is nowhere more apparent than in the evaluation process.

When all goes well, evaluation is a mutually congratulatory experience that enhances the confidence of supervisor and supervisee. When the intern's progress is not evident, it is much harder. It is difficult to criticize and make someone else unhappy; yet learning problems must be identified and openly discussed. When supervisors feel uncomfortable being open about the intern's learning problems, it is helpful to keep in mind how much more difficulty will arise if they postpone the discussion. The earlier learning issues are raised, the less possibility there is of a defensive response.

When professional schools place interns in community and institutional settings, they appoint a liaison to insure that school and field are working together. Academic workloads may be great and school advisors may not always reach out to the supervisor. It is thus important and appropriate for the supervisor who is faced with a problematic situation to reach out to the school advisor for advice and support. If such an encounter is unavailable or unsatisfactory, someone further up in the school's chain of command can be contacted. As the agency supervisor has a responsibility to the school, the school also has a responsibility to the agency supervisor. Neither the agency supervisor nor the school can educate the intern to be an effective practitioner without the help of the other.

Part V:
Supervising Direct Care Workers

Chapter 14

Shared Tasks and Issues

We use the term "direct care worker" to describe paraprofessional workers who help dependent older people with activities of daily living. In the home of the older person, they may be known as home health aides, home care workers, or companions. In an assisted living or nursing home facility, they may be known as nursing assistants or companions.

The relationship between the elder and the direct care worker is by its very nature intensely close and personal. Both have common goals: the elder can only function with a provider compensating for the losses that make it impossible to manage independently; the caregiver's employment is dependent on the care and well-being of the elder. At the same time, issues of mistrust occur on both sides, and cultural and socioeconomic differences can make these relationships fraught with anxiety and disappointment.

Supervising direct care workers is a very different process from supervising professional workers. However, it is our contention that

Gerontological Supervision
© 2008 by The Haworth Press, Taylor & Francis Group. All rights reserved.
doi:10.1300/5153_14

the social work model of supervision can be translated to this group and used effectively to enhance the caring relationship.

TASKS

Whether they work in the older person's own home or in a residential facility, direct care workers have common tasks, such as helping with bathing, dressing, toileting, and feeding to a greater or lesser extent depending on the elder's needs and wishes. However, the work settings, hours, other responsibilities, and work conditions are dissimilar—posing different issues for the supervisor.

In the Home

Home care workers also have responsibilities for light housekeeping, food shopping, escorting, and household chores. They may spend anywhere from four to twenty-four hours a day alone with a single older person and are the agency representatives on-site charged with noting and reporting changes that occur in elder functioning. Co-workers and supervisors are off-site.

In a Residential Facility

Certified nursing assistants in residential facilities also make beds, select clothing (hopefully with the resident), and escort clients to appointments and activities. They are responsible for six to twelve older people depending on the shift, giving each thirty minutes to one hour of attention. Co-workers and supervisors are on-site.

ISSUES

There are differences and similarities between care providers depending on the setting.

Intimacy

The relationship between the elder and the care provider is intensely intimate. The care provider performs functions that all of us past the toddler stage handle ourselves in private. However, home care workers provide personal care in the privacy of the elder's home. Privacy is a goal, not a reality in most nursing homes and care is commonly provided in "tub rooms," common toilet areas, or behind a drawn curtain. Intimacy for the elder often encompasses many more people, including other nursing assistants, unit staff, roommates, and other residents, any of whom may witness any aspect of care including toileting.

Cultural Differences

Elders and direct care workers commonly come from different cultural backgrounds. Often both parties come with stereotypical beliefs. Racial comments by the cognitively compromised elder can be offensive to a care provider. A lack of interest in the care and handling of kosher food by a care provider can engender mistrust in the elder.

Cultural differences often result in the firing and replacing of care providers by the elderly in their own homes. Nursing assistants in a nursing home setting have the advantage of their numbers. Responsibilities can be adjusted so that a care provider is better able to deal with offensive comments and care for the disinhibited elder.

Work Hours

Home care providers commonly work long hours. When the elder is cognitively impaired or otherwise dependent for assistance in all or most activities of daily living, these shifts may extend for twelve or twenty-four hours at a time. However, not every moment is spent providing care and days can be long and boring for the direct care workers. At the same time, elders often resent paying for someone to "sit around and do nothing." Assistants in nursing homes have many patients to care for, and multiple demands and tasks. They are often criticized by the elderly and their families for not responding in a timely manner. In addition, they have documentation requirements, which is almost never the case for home care workers.

Workplace Issues

The job of a direct care worker is a low status position. The pay is minimal, the status is among the lowest for legitimate positions and there is no upward mobility. Because of their more intense relationship with clients and families, direct care workers typically receive more credit and gratification, but make less money and have no job security. A home care provider may lose her job and income if the elder she is caring for dies or is hospitalized. Or she may randomly be removed from a case and assigned to a new client by the agency. Assistants in nursing homes have job security and are better paid and trained, but have the least status in the community at large.

Accountability

The elder and/or the elder's family employ direct care workers. The employer is not always aware of how to evaluate care. Obviously a care provider with a good attendance record and positive interaction with the client will be evaluated positively. However, the thoroughness of the care provided may not be evaluated or even considered by the employer. Nursing assistants, on the other hand, are commonly evaluated on very objective criteria. However, positive interactions and feedback may not be considered significant, or even relevant, by the assistant's supervisor.

Using a social work practice model of supervision would result in better care as the provider learns and grows in the role. As the opportunity to work out difficulties between the provider and elder is present, it is likely that the provider will stay in one position for a longer period of time, resulting in better and more cost-effective service. This model will unquestionably result in higher satisfaction on both sides.

Chapter 15

Home Care

DIRECT CARE IN THE COMMUNITY

Although terms may vary from state to state (or even from agency to agency), direct care workers who work in the home of the older person have different levels of training and responsibility.

The Home Health Aide

Home health aides work under the direction of a nurse and can administer oral medications as well as provide hands-on care. Home health aides take temperatures, and check pulse rates, assist in all activities of daily living and change nonsterile dressings. They take a competency test (federal requirement) to be certified. Training is offered in trade schools and community colleges. The training covers the common nursing procedures, such as how to read a thermometer, take a pulse, and what to document. Training is helpful in passing the test, but not required.

The Home Care Worker

Home care workers provide largely nonmedical care such as housekeeping and routine personal care. Home care workers clean house, do laundry, shop, and cook for the care of the elderly. They may also help clients out of bed, assist with bathing, dressing and grooming, and accompany an elder to an appointment or activity. There are no formal requirements or training for a home care worker.

Gerontological Supervision
© 2008 by The Haworth Press, Taylor & Francis Group. All rights reserved.
doi:10.1300/5153_15

Companions

Companions are not required to have any formal training and (at least theoretically) they provide only for nonmedical/physical needs such as reading, letter writing, and escorting to appointments or activities. In reality, companions often provide hands-on care under the direction of the elderly person and/or the family. Companions are generally paid less.

SUPERVISION OF HOME CARE WORKERS

A case manager is often the supervisor of the home care worker in the field. They both might share a supervisor back at the office. Having a peer as well as hierarchal relationship in relation to the agency, knowing clients in their home environments, and sharing their idiosyncrasies and concerns, generally produces a good working relationship.

ASSESSING STRENGTHS AND UNCOVERING POSSIBLE PROBLEMS

Supervision for home care workers is practical and problem focused. The supervisor needs to begin with an assessment of the care provider so that she or he can identify and use strengths already existent, as well as uncover possible problem areas. Although it is not feasible to think in terms of a forty-five minute one-on-one supervision with providers, the initial meeting should allow for a private conversation to gather enough information for an assessment.

Sarah, the case manager, met Alison, the care provider at Mrs. Caly's home, where she was assigned work for twelve hours five days a week. Sarah noted Alison's cheerful demeanor as well as her high energy evidenced by the freshly scrubbed floor in the kitchen and just-baked brownies on the table. Asked about her background, Alison talked about her experience in child welfare commenting on the sadness in the lives of many children and how uncaring many parents are. Called by Mrs. Caly, Alison rolled her eyes as she explained that Mrs. Caly had already had lunch. When Mrs. Caly insisted she was starving, Alison spelled out what she had eaten for lunch. Alison asked Sarah if there was a limit on how many calls from Mrs. Caly's daughter she had to respond to as she felt that the daughter called just to check that she was there.

From this conversation Sarah could gauge many strengths. Alison is hardworking, responsive, and energetic. Although her background gave her skills in provision of care, she had no knowledge of the elderly or dementia. She could also see that difficulties with parents in child welfare may have led to fear and mistrust of Mrs. Caly's family.

Sarah explained her role as case manager and spelled out clearly that supervision of Alison's handling of Mrs. Caly's care was part of her job. She commended Alison on how well Mrs. Caly looks and how clean she keeps the kitchen. She presented some strategies for handling dementia in the elderly, suggesting that distracting Mrs. Caly when she wants lunch again will be more successful than arguing with her. She also shared the recent past of the Caly's family. The previous care provider had left Mrs. Caly alone on two occasions. She said that Alison should anticipate frequent calls until the daughter begins to trust Alison. She suggested that Alison take the initiative when the daughter called by telling her an event of the day, such as she had just made brownies for an afternoon treat. Sarah told her that it is likely the calls will decrease when the daughter is assured, but, if not, Alison should let her know and she would meet with the daughter.

Sarah noted that future meetings should focus on learning skills to work with elders with dementia, and helping Alison understand family fears and expectations.

RESPONDING NOT REACTING

Developing a sense of professional identity is also helpful in dealing with common problems of the elderly. Angry outbursts on the part of a confused older person are common, and attempts to leave the premises ("I am late for work." "I have to pick up Paula from school.") are also frequent challenging moments. Direct care workers who have learned to respond rather than react will not panic. Instead they will be able to intervene effectively at the moment. Telling an old person they have no business yelling will not help. Instead asking the elder what happened to make them so upset will. Assuring a frightened older person that she is not late for work and asking about her office routine will calm her down. Explaining that an old man has been retired for thirty years will exacerbate an already problematic situation.

CULTURAL/ETHNIC DIFFERENCES

Confounding factors in the provider/receiver relationship is the cultural divide between them. Cultural/ethnic differences are commonly a part of this complicated relationship and can significantly affect it. Racial and ethnic sensitivity is highlighted in our culture, and both sides can potentially use and abuse ethnic differences.

Mrs. Hayes routinely complained to her African-American caregiver about the deterioration of her neighborhood since blacks had replaced most of the Irish. She also frequently accused her of stealing ("like all of you people") items she had misplaced. Her caregiver, Elsie, grumbled under her breath at these attacks and tried to ignore them. She did make a point to Mrs. Hayes, and often in the presence of Mrs. Hayes' son and daughter-in-law, that her people do not hire others to care for their elderly.

Negative cultural/racial issues can impact severely on the relationship between a homebound client and her direct care worker. One successful intervention is to work with both parties about the underlying issues. When Mrs. Hayes uses racial stereotypes about theft, what is she trying to articulate? The case manager can validate and share the feelings of anger, but work with the care provider around the underlying feeling. She can also help the provider understand her underlying anger when she talks about her people "caring for their own."

CM: "You must feel very angry with both Mrs. Hayes and her family."

ELSIE: "I don't let it bother me."

CM: "When you say your people don't hire strangers to care for their elderly, it sounds to me like you are mad."

ELSIE: "We don't, and if she weren't so mean, they might take care of her like they should."

CM: "She can be mean, but can you think of reasons why?"

ELSIE: "She doesn't like to have help. She wants to do everything herself and she cries when she can't."

Similarly a discussion with the elder and her family about how it feels to be accused of theft and some education about other cultures can be effective. Once again both sides should be offered alternative providers and clients. However, the emphasis needs to be on the problems, which will not disappear if they opt for a change.

The case manager for Elsie and Mrs. Hayes met with Mrs. Hayes and her daughter to discuss how things were going. She asked both to indicate what is going well. The daughter said that Elsie is reliable and hard working. She takes good care of the house and of Mrs. Hayes. Mrs. Hayes reluctantly agreed. The case manager commented that it is hard to have someone in your home when you are used to being on your own. She asked how they think it is for Elsie when she is accused of stealing. Mrs. Hayes said, "She knows I am joking." The case manager said she was not so sure that Elsie took it as a joke. She discussed the meaning of personal integrity in the Island culture. Mrs. Hayes' daughter said it is similar to the strong personal honesty of those from the west of Ireland.

Interventions with these challenging issues are ongoing and problems are not solved in one session. However, incremental change to more positive interactions is a very likely outcome with this kind of ongoing supervision.

Helping a direct care worker depersonalize racial or ethnic slurs is an important supervisory intervention. In the culture that we live in, these kinds of insults are especially inflammatory. Education about cognitive loss, disinhibition, and the cultural background of the elder is helpful. It is also useful to point out that these kinds of insults speak to the helplessness and loss of control that the elder is experiencing.

Elena, home care worker for Mrs. Henderson, called her supervisor from a coffee shop to tell her she had been fired again. Mrs. Henderson had called her a "dirty spic" and ordered her off the premises. Her supervisor asked what had caused the upset. Elena said that Mrs. Henderson had decided to shower alone and had almost slipped. Elena had been hiding behind the door and grabbed her in time. During and after the shower, Mrs. Henderson had berated her. The supervisor asked what the next steps might be. What was the motto for Mrs. Henderson? Elena sighed and said "Respond, don't react!" "What happens next?" the supervisor asked. "I am on my way back to tell her she can't fire me because she needs me and let's watch 'As the World Turns.'" The supervisor laughed and said, "Tell her you are too lazy to work anyway."

In this example, the supervisor is careful to not overreact. First, she got the full story. Giving Elena the opportunity to relay the story is also a way of helping her solve her problem. This is not the first time that this kind of upset has occurred and the supervisor reminded Elena that she knows what to do. Joking with her about racial stereotypes was also an effective way of minimizing personal hurt. Helping direct care workers learn how to respond and not react allows them to build a strong professional identity.

INTIMACY ISSUES

Intimacy issues are probably the greatest challenge for care providers and their clients. It is not surprising that fecal incontinence is the primary reason for nursing home placement. Caring family members often provide heroic service in the care of an elderly relative. Experienced geriatricians are familiar with stories of daughters who travel hours every day to shop and cook for a parent, or families who devote weekends and free time to the care of a relative. Assisting with household chores can be a given in many families, and families with financial means typically pay for household help for the elder. Incontinence is typically the breaking point for families in terms of their comfort level in providing care and supporting the elder in the community. Intimate care is almost universally provided by strangers, which will increase the anxiety of even a significantly demented elder. Elders often complain about "rough" treatment. Intervening in what can possibly be abuse is an enormous challenge for the case manager.

Karen, case manager for a day program, received a call from Mrs. Hardy's daughter. She told Karen that her mother complained that her new care provider treated her meanly and was rough when she changed her. Karen asked the program nurse to examine Mrs. Hardy. With no apparent injury, Karen then spoke to Mrs. Hardy who spoke fondly of her former care provider and negatively about all aspects of the care offered by her new provider. Karen encouraged the discussion about the former worker, asking if she remembered how she felt when she first had a care provider. Mrs. Hardy recognized that she had some discomfort initially with her first caregiver, but insisted that Sharon, her current provider, is a mean person. Karen was aware that Sharon had a good record in the five years she worked for the agency. She talked to Sharon openly about Mrs. Hardy's complaints and allowed her to ventilate about her difficulties. She was also aware that Sharon had one client for almost four years until her sudden death six months ago. Karen realized that both parties in this relationship were mourning. She talked with Sharon about how hard it is to begin with a new client and then worked with her about how she can begin to establish rapport with Mrs. Hardy. As a part of her discussion with Sharon and Mrs. Hardy she offered both a change in assignment, but strongly encouraged them both to give this relationship a chance. Both were willing and Karen devoted significant time to working with Sharon on how to intervene effectively, and not person-alize some of Mrs. Hardy's responses.

In this example, Karen's first intervention is crucial. A report of abuse or mistreatment must be investigated and physical and/or verbal abuse ruled out. The next step is an assessment of both parties. In this case, it is clear that emotional issues on both sides were a big part of the problem. There could also have been a misunderstanding of the home care role on the part of the client or the family.

Another key element of Karen's intervention is offering a change of assignment to both. Both elders and care providers often feel pow-erless in the world they live in. Offering a change gives both parties a sense of control, and frees them to choose to stay together and work on establishing rapport.

INDIVIDUALIZING THE CLIENT

Home care offers the personal care assistant the opportunity to in-dividualize the client. Times for meals, bathing, and recreation can be tailored to his particular preferences and routines. Long hours alone together foster a form of intimacy not possible in a residential setting where shift changes and full workloads are the norm. The intimacy be-tween client and worker fosters leeway for the worker as well. When clients view direct care workers as "one of the family" boundaries can become blurred—often outside the knowledge of the case manager or supervisor. So it is that the direct care worker with financial problems may borrow money from the client that she has no ability to pay back. Or the client and direct care worker may share "secrets" about trun-cated work hours or noncompliance with medication regimes that the medical team believes are being followed. Thus a relationship where there are no expressed complaints on either side may raise ethical or practice concerns even when there is no question of the client's men-tal competence. In the presence of cognitive impairment, the dangers are greater. Interviewing the client when the home care worker is not present provides an opportunity to explore these less tangible aspects of the relationship.

Chapter 16

Residential Care

DIRECT CARE IN THE NURSING HOME

Nursing home nursing assistants must be certified before they can work in long-term care. Certified nursing assistants are required to take a hundred-hour course which trains them in the physical care of the residents as well as providing some information on emotional needs and dementia. They work under the direct supervision of an RN or LPN. Typically, nursing assistants have a series of tasks to be completed in a time span (shift). They care for a cluster of residents, providing assistance with basic care (transferring in and out of bed and wheelchair, personal hygiene, dressing, toileting, bathing, and feeding).

THE INSTITUTIONAL MODEL

Long-term care is traditionally provided in an institutional model. Residents eat, bathe, and are toileted on a schedule not necessarily related to the resident's needs or wishes, but rather to the institution's time frame. The institutional model usually results in dissatisfaction on both sides. Nursing assistants and nurses who work the night shift express feelings of sadness and guilt that they are required to wake up some residents, provide morning care, and get them out of bed before the start of the day shift. Residents and their families will express dissatisfaction about "long waits" for care while a nursing assistant is busy caring for other residents.

In the institutional model, care planning is usually done by the professional staff with little or no input by the assistants, and nursing assistants are seldom included in discussions about discharge planning

Gerontological Supervision
© 2008 by The Haworth Press, Taylor & Francis Group. All rights reserved.
doi:10.1300/5153_16

for residents, electing palliative care, or transfers to specialized units—even though they usually know more about the residents' needs and wishes than other staff. The institutional model, therefore, promotes a sense of powerlessness among the nursing assistants and residents which often results in exacerbating negative interactions between these two groups.

The culture of long-term care makes it challenging, but not impossible, to intervene effectively using a social work supervisory model.

Greg is a community coordinator in a nursing home whose role is to direct the care on one unit with all staff reporting to him. Lucy, the CNA, is on the phone trying to reach a Union delegate as Mr. Weaver, a resident on that floor with moderate dementia has accused her of stealing his wristwatch. Greg asks Lucy to talk to him in his office. Lucy is obviously distraught, feeling threatened, and at risk of losing her good reputation after fifteen years of service to the home. Assuring her that he knows she would never steal from anyone, he talks in terms of Mr. Weaver's fears about his declining cognitive status and his history of accusing others when he forgets where he puts things. Greg suggested they could think of Mr. Weaver's certainty that he never loses or forgets anything as a strength, even though it is inconvenient for the staff. Greg suggested that they both go to his room and look for the watch. Greg suggested that Lucy assure him that she wants to help solve a problem when he accuses her again.

Greg, as the supervisor, demonstrates support for Lucy to reduce her fear and anxiety, as he educates her about cognitive loss and helps to work out a plan to solve the problem. Even with an impeccable record, Lucy's first response to an accusation is fear and defensiveness. Greg knows this nursing assistant, but what if he did not know her so well? How does he then investigate a complaint, work with the assistant, and respect the rights and feelings of the resident? The task in these situations is quite formidable. However, even when the situation is not so clear, it is still important to hold to the agreed upon model of supervision.

Greg would still talk to the assistant and listen carefully to what happened. He would also talk to the resident and engage both in a process of searching for the lost item. If the item was not found, as the coordinator of the unit, he would use available resources (log books or valuables lists) to ascertain that the watch was on the premises. He would also investigate among staff and residents when the item was last seen. Depending on agency policy, he might replace the item or reimburse with money. He would have to both reassure the nursing assistant and be mindful of the complaint in the event of any future incidents.

CONFLICTING PHILOSOPHIES OF CARE

In large, long-term care facilities that offer services ranging from subacute to terminal care it is not uncommon to find conflicting philosophies of care.

David, a hospice social worker, has a patient who needs nursing home placement; because of bed unavailability, the patient is on a rehab floor. The patient is complaining bitterly that she is forced out of bed and "encouraged to eat" no matter how nauseous she is. He asks to meet with the care team and is surprised that the nursing assistant is not there. He strongly encourages her participation and the team agrees. They meet and review the care expectations for a hospice resident. David is careful to let the head nurse confirm that a hospice patient can stay in bed, and eat when and if they want to. He brings in an aide from the hospice program to meet with the nursing assistants caring for this patient so that they can communicate directly about what the expectations are.

Long-term care facilities are only beginning to learn how to better use their resources and staff. The advantages of getting and giving information to the hands-on caregiver are obvious, but not always understood in nursing facilities. It was important in this example that David understood the importance of having the nurse validate his discussion about hospice care. It was also helpful to bring in a peer from his program to work with the nursing assistant.

HANDLING RESIDENT/FAMILY COMPLAINTS

Nursing assistants are frequently the targets of resident/family complaints. Many older people and their families come to long-term care fearing poor treatment or abuse. Media coverage frequently encourages these preconceived notions. Nursing assistants are commonly fearful of complaints that will reflect negatively on their ability to retain their positions or to receive pay increases. Both sides, therefore, approach each other with suspicion and mistrust. Intervention for the case manager is complicated by the fact that nursing assistants can be, at the very least, thoughtless in approach. Common complaints from residents/ families include nursing assistants performing tasks without interacting with the resident, two nursing assistants talking to each other while providing care, and assistants complaining to residents and families about staffing and overwork. Nursing assistants complain that families ignore them, and then go to higher ups without first bringing a problem to their attention.

Susan, a long-term care social worker, was surprised to hear a complaint from a new resident's family about Ms. Linton, a nursing assistant with many years of experience and a reputation as a caring person. The complaint was that she was rude, manifested in not responding to questions, and not speaking to either the resident or the family. When she asked Ms. Linton, she reported that she had heard through the grapevine that the family were VIP's and would get special treatment. She was afraid of saying the wrong thing. Susan talked to her about the number of residents and families she had worked with over the years. She also mentioned that all patients are "VIP" people, who want what we all want for our elderly relatives. Susan assured her that she would work well with them if she were just herself.

CULTURAL/ETHNIC DIFFERENCE

Cultural and ethnic differences also present challenges in residential care. As discussed in Chapter 15, differences in expectations on both sides, anger at the place of direct care workers and the frail elderly in this society, disinhibited elderly clients, and stereotypical thinking can result in anger and hostility between direct care workers and their clients.

Rhonda, nurse manager on a subacute floor, received a complaint about Sheila, a nursing assistant, from a newly admitted resident. Sheila was a nurse from Ireland who was working as a nursing assistant while waiting to get licensed as a nurse. The new resident was Hispanic, but fluent in English. Her complaint was that Sheila favored white residents and ignored her. She also said that Sheila was quick and abrupt when "forced" to care for her.

Rhonda asked Sheila about her new residents. In discussing the Hispanic resident, Sheila mentioned that she has trouble understanding her, even though her English is good. Rhonda said that the resident felt that she discriminated against her. Sheila said that was a very unfair thing to say. She said she treats everyone the same. This particular resident is able and needs to be encouraged to be more independent. Rhonda asked whether encouraging independence might be misunderstood by the resident. Sheila thought about this and said she does avoid this resident because it is embarrassing to keep asking her to repeat what she says. Sheila said that she would talk with her and acknowledge that they needed to work together to understand each other.

In this example, the resident assumed that Sheila discriminated because she avoided her. Sheila assumed that since the resident was cognitively intact and able to make her needs known, it did not matter. Both sides misinterpreted the behavior of the other. Rhonda offered suggestions, rather than accusations. She allowed Sheila to think about what she was doing. Sheila was then able to acknowledge her own discomfort with this resident, and reach out to the resident to establish a working relationship.

HANDLING SEXUALITY AND BODILY FUNCTIONS

Institutional care, as mentioned earlier, limits privacy for even the most personal issues. Residents are forced to accept being wheeled to a shower room wrapped in a towel. Old facilities may not allow for a bathroom door to close when an aide is helping a resident use the toilet. Roommates and visitors smell a resident who has just had his or her brief changed behind a pulled curtain. Any kind of sexual expression can evoke shock or amusement among staff and other residents.

The nurse case manager noticed snickering among the staff about Mr. Miller who had just been admitted to a long-term floor. The evening staff had twice observed him masturbating when they entered his room. She engaged the staff in a discussion about rights and privacy, suggesting that all of us do things in the privacy of our home, which we would not want observed by others. She reminded staff that if they knock and do not get a reply, they could come back later. She also reminded them that closing the door and respecting his privacy, rather than snickering, was the more appropriate intervention.

Issues are seldom this clear. Residents have the right to sexual expression between themselves, but this right also opens up issues of privacy, informed consent, and the involvement of other residents and the individuals' families. Consenting adults can certainly make their own decisions about sexual contact. However, in semiprivate rooms, the rights of the roommate have to be respected as well. Residents may have some capacity to select partners, but not necessarily have full capacity. Staff and families need to be involved in discussion in such situations with the understanding that the wishes and life patterns of the residents involved will be primary in determining how the agency will assist the residents in freedom of expression.

Some facilities offer privacy rooms where people can spend time together. Sometimes residents work out systems not unlike what many of us experienced in college in terms of negotiations with roommates. Long-term care is a very complicated world where the rights of the individual versus the rights of the group creates an ongoing dialogue among staff, residents, and families.

Elisa, the social worker on a nursing floor with a relatively high function-ing population, came in on Monday to a scandal on her floor. Mr. White had been in the room of a new resident, Ms. Sanders. The couple had been having sexual contact on her bed. Many residents on the unit were shocked. Staff was at a loss as to what to do. As team leader, Elisa called a staff meeting first. They reviewed the charts and determined that Ms. Sanders had capacity. Mr. White could make his own choices in many areas, but had a dementia diagnosis. Elisa then met with both parties and explained that sexual contact had to be in a place that was private and that Elisa would work to establish a private place. She then contacted Mr. White's son and reviewed the situation with him. He agreed that his father can make a decision about how he social-izes and was not being exploited. As other residents approached her, she re-iterated that her job is to make sure that rights are protected and that people have privacy. She then discussed two options with her supervisor. They could offer to move the couple together or offer one a private room. She then re-viewed the options with the unit staff and with the couple. Ms. Sanders was ultimately offered a private room.

FLEXIBILITY WITHIN JOB REQUIREMENTS

Aggressive behavior can also be exacerbated by an institutional setting. Long-term care residents commonly will be aggressive when pushed to do something they do not want to do. At home with one-on-one care, home care workers are more comfortable with a flexible schedule. In the nursing home, the task orientation is often primary. Nursing assistants will push to have a shower at eleven-o'clock and this insistence can lead to verbal and physical aggression on the part of the resident.

Nursing assistants who want to do a good job may interpret their work schedule rigidly—always tackling tasks in a particular order. Sometimes a colleague can suggest a modification that responds to a resident's individual needs without sacrificing time. (Such common problems are also useful topics for group supervision.)

Ms. Grey, an experienced nursing assistant, helped her colleague who was unsuccessfully trying to persuade Mrs. Chambers that it was indeed Tuesday, that she hadn't just had a shower, and no she could not take a shower after the Johnny Carson show because Johnny Carson had died a long time ago. Ms. Grey was able to convince her colleague not to discuss Johnny Carson's funeral. She suggested instead that she leave Mrs. Chambers to her television, give Mrs. Handel a shower (since she is always ready), and try Mrs. Chambers later. Ms. Grey assured her that in the long run, she could guarantee that she was saving, not losing, time.

Chapter 17

Group Supervision, Training, and Evaluation

GROUP SUPERVISION

Group supervision is a highly effective way of enhancing skills and helping direct care workers to learn from each other. Some settings, nursing homes, home care agencies, and day programs, for example, have many providers in one location. In these settings, groups are both possible and practical. Groups allow each member to support each other as well as share knowledge and problems. As members get acquainted, they become increasingly comfortable asking for help and support. Group supervision can also be very beneficial in a long-term care setting.

HANDLING CHALLENGING SITUATIONS

Nursing assistants who have the opportunity to express their positive and negative feelings about their job experience significant relief from stress and feel valued and understood. Nursing assistants can also benefit from the experiences of their peers in handling challenging situations.

Ellen, nurse supervisor in a long-term facility, meets regularly with the nurses and the aides she supervises. At her meeting with the nursing assistants, they focused on a family considered very "demanding." Ellen encouraged ventilating of feelings, assured them that the family was going to have

Gerontological Supervision
© 2008 by The Haworth Press, Taylor & Francis Group. All rights reserved.
doi:10.1300/5153_17

to be a part of their unit and helped them discuss ways they had managed other problem families in the past. One assistant suggested letting each of them take a turn at caring for the resident and letting the family select the regular aide. The group enjoyed the thought of a contest where the winner loses. However, they also agreed that this family would probably be more content with whomever they selected.

DISCUSSING POLICY CHANGES

Group meetings can be a good vehicle to communicate and get feedback on policy changes. However, announcements are not the right choice when it comes to effective communication. Groups are only effective when everyone is listening and communicating. A policy change should engender a discussion and appropriate feedback should be brought to the policy makers.

The evening nurse supervisor met with the nursing staff. There was a directive from the State about documenting food intake that she needed to discuss. She read the directive to the staff and asked for comments. When no one said anything, she commented that the directive was broad and they had to work on how to implement it successfully. She further explained that the State wanted only the outcome, it was up to them to figure out how to make it work, preferably by using their existing documentation. The prospect of complying without additional work engendered a lot of interest and discussion.

TEASING OUT SUCCESSFUL INTERVENTIONS

The supervisor plays a key role in facilitating group interaction and particularly in sifting through the discussion to tease out successful interventions.

Jane, a social worker in a nonprofit home care agency, meets with a group of aides on Wednesday evenings when they pick up their paychecks. The contract for this group is to share the struggles that they have with their patients and help each other learn skills to improve their techniques. At this meeting, Jane listened carefully as Wanda recounted her difficulty getting her patient to take a shower. Many colleagues experienced similar problems and shared their experiences. Jane asked the group to help her identify successful interventions. Thinking together they agreed that not insisting and agreeing to another time, worked sometimes. They also agreed that at times the prospect of a visit from a family member is an incentive. One aide stated that she sets things up and leaves her patient alone in the bath with the door ajar in case of a problem. Jane pointed out that sometimes you just can not persuade a confused elderly person and suggested that they keep in mind that no one ever died from missing an occasional bath.

At another meeting Jane listened to Helen talk about how she understands her aphasic patient. She asked Helen how she figured out what she was trying to say. Helen said that initially she watched Mrs. King's eyes and tried to respond quickly so that Mrs. King did not get frustrated. When she was right they were both happy. When Helen was wrong, she made fun of herself and said that Mrs. King was stuck with a beginner. Helen commented, "People can laugh with their eyes." Jane pointed out how Helen eliminated the frustration and agitation, which are typical symptoms with poststroke patients. Another care provider mentioned that frustration and agitation makes everything worse anyway and all agreed. Jane mentioned Helen was also able to learn from her patient by watching her eyes and understanding what she was looking for. She talked with the group about what kind of nonverbal cues can be understood and how much easier that can make the job.

PROVIDING EMOTIONAL SUPPORT FOR MEMBERS

Groups can also provide emotional support for members:

The night supervisor in a nursing home met with the aides on each floor routinely. When she arrived on one Friday at midnight, Mrs. Schaeffer was very quiet. When asked what was wrong, she talked about how she spoke to Mrs. Ronan last night when she woke up, about her new great granddaughter. When she came in this evening, Mrs. Ronan had died so unexpectedly. In addition, there was a new resident in the bed. Mrs. Schaeffer said, "I know it is not the new resident's fault, but I felt so close to Mrs. Ronan." The group talked about the sadness of loss. They also talked about how hard it is to work nights and be so separated from the events and changes that occur every day.

A less than confident facilitator may legitimately be reluctant to meet his or her supervisees in a group. There is safety in numbers, and there is a risk (and a hope for outcome) that the group may challenge the leader.

At a meeting with the day program director, the staff was very quiet. He commented on the silence which continued. He asked if someone could tell him what was wrong. Someone finally mentioned the afternoon program.

After some hesitation, someone said that he wanted a larger number of participants which they all understood. However, the new members arrived when they had formerly done paperwork. Now there is no time for paper work. The director listened and acknowledged that he should have talked with the staff first. He apologized and asked if they could help figure out how to make all this work. After a lengthy discussion, they decided that half the staff could greet and settle the new members while the others did paper work. They would cut back on one group so that the other half could take some paper time later in the afternoon.

The Importance of "Rambling"

Although it is important to keep to an agreed upon time, supervisors should be comfortable letting a discussion "ramble" if everyone is engaged. Direct care work is often a very isolating experience (especially in the community) and the opportunity to share similar life experiences can be very gratifying to the care providers. Direct care workers are often not aware of how very skilled they are, and benefit enormously when their intuitive ability is identified and named.

TRAINING

A Specific Focus

Every individual or group supervisory experience is training. However, training with a specific focus (caring for the diabetic patient, understanding Alzheimer's disease) can be a very rewarding experience for care workers. Like a group, training offers the providers the chance to be together and to learn. The knowledge gained also has a secondary gain in promoting a sense of professionalism among providers. One author recently had the experience of interviewing a nursing assistant who had been through customer service training. The nursing assistant was very enthusiastic about a problem solving method she learned in the class and was quite articulate in her plans to implement her new problem solving skills in her interaction with a very fussy family member. She also said she felt so inspired by what she learned that she was considering going back to school.

PROMOTING WORKER INVOLVEMENT
AND COMFORT

Training sessions will typically feature speakers on relevant topics. It is helpful to include care workers in decisions about what kind of training is offered. Problems related to the health of the elderly are common topics. In addition, such topics as infection control, nail care, and alternative bathing techniques are popular topics. Psychosocial issues, such as elder abuse, alcoholism in the elderly, and challenging families, are also relevant. Teaching communication skills and how to work cooperatively, if done well, are also very effective.

Training should be ongoing in that the learning is not only topic related, but is also significantly correlated with high morale and promoting professionalism. Obviously there is a cost to training. Topic information, speakers, and videos all cost money. In addition, the providers must be replaced in some instances and paid for their time. However, the benefits are significant and areas such as customer satisfaction, increase in referrals, and staff retention have to be considered. Training is commonly well worth its costs.

Supervisors of direct care workers need to be alert to the comfort level of the staff in training classes and in everyday communication. Literacy in English varies greatly in this population. It is often helpful to ask what is easiest for the care worker: "Shall I leave you a voice mail or is a note better?" In training classes, supervisors need to be alert to any discomfort among participants. It is important to ask for volunteers if anything needs to be read out loud.

EVALUATION

Direct care workers typically experience evaluations negatively. They are perceived as threatening, potentially resulting in loss of income and positions. Even very good workers will focus only on the negatives aspects of an evaluation if they are not involved in the process.

Preparation and Discussion

A successful evaluation process begins with preparation and discussion. The supervisor should show the supervisee the evaluation document and talk about what both will bring to the conference. The workers should be encouraged to discuss what they do well, and what areas need to be improved upon.

When the supervisor and supervisee meet, the supervisor should focus on helping the worker articulate what she or he does well and why and what areas need improvement. The supervisor may need to give examples to clarify or ask probing questions. This is not a process that comes easily to nonsocial workers and will be a challenge to the supervisor. However, this process is worth the difficulty as workers begin to "own" their strengths and weaknesses and utilize what they learn.

Evaluations for workers cover both the concrete services provided and the ability to work with the elder and the elder's family. A nursing assistant in a nursing home will be evaluated on understanding infection control policies and procedures, ability to get ADL tasks accomplished in a designated time frame, documentation, attendance, and use of sick time. All are reasonable criteria. However, skills in engaging and understanding the elderly, and ability to work with families should also be part of an evaluation. Home care workers are typically evaluated (if at all) using similar criteria. Evaluations are done by the supervisor and usually based on questioning the provider and reviewing documentation as well as attendance records.

The Evaluation Tool

Using the social work perspective as outlined earlier would incorporate all of the above criteria, but also focus on enhancing and building interpersonal skills. An evaluation tool might include communication skills, dependability, initiative, cooperation, and compliance with regulations. The supervisor might assess some areas by engaging in a dialogue with the supervisee.

Ruth, social work manager at a home care agency, met with Angie, home attendant for Mrs. Blake, for her annual evaluation. Angie had been with the agency for four years and Mrs. Blake was her third patient. Ruth asked how this relatively new assignment was working. Angie said it had been hard in the beginning, but that she had observed Mrs. Blake as much as possible and could now better predict her needs and wishes. Angie mentioned how much she had learned over the years. She said that training on dementia had helped her so much, and she no longer got angry when yelled at. Also, she could understand more quickly how to reassure people and the work was much smoother. From this discussion, Ruth could see that Angie had advanced in terms of appropriate communication. In addition, she paid attention during learning opportunities and used skills that she had learned.

In other instances, a supervisor can uncover and identify areas for improvement during the coming year:

Carol is the care coordinator on a nursing home unit. Among her supervisees is Serena, a nursing assistant. Serena has been with the home for three years. Evaluations have indicated that she is adequate, but not outstanding. Carol raised with her some complaints from the evening staff about tasks left undone from Serena's cluster of residents. Serena insisted that she had too much work and could not possibly get her work done most days. She pointed out that Mrs. Marney's daughter was there most days and micromanaged every thing Serena did. Asked how she handles this problem, Serena said she stops working and calls the nurse. Carol asked if that works and Serena said "no."

Carol asked her to think of what might work, suggesting that the daughter might do better if Serena greeted her and updated her in the morning. Serena was sure that would not work, but agreed that she would try. From this discussion, Carol could see that Serena was both rigid and fearful. The evaluation noted her need to bring problems to her supervisor before they got too difficult and the need for in-service education on communication to help Serena advance.

The evaluation should be a learning tool. Clear, understandable goals for the coming year should be a part of the evaluation, and both players should work toward achieving them.

Afterword

Social work has long been a leader in the theory of strength-based supervision. In practice, however, many case management and long-term care settings view supervision as a purely administrative function: "top down" directives with emphasis on compliance with agency directives rather than a participatory encounter in which practitioners can learn and grow on the job.

It is our hope that a social work perspective will be utilized extensively in community services and long-term care settings to create workers on every level with the knowledge and skills necessary to provide better service to an elderly and typically vulnerable population. Although there are discipline specific knowledge and skills, the principles of social work supervision are universally applicable. Highlighting strengths and crediting abilities will always enhance a worker's morale. Identifying areas in need of improvement before a crisis, discussing openly what obstacles are apparent, and suggesting alternate interventions will always make any worker feel empowered and more independent. Addressing an ineffective intervention and focusing on looking at more effective ways to help will always make a worker feel secure and valued.

Although the social work perspective is effective, even committed and experienced supervisors will not always use it. Errors in judgment, negative countertransference, and off days will always occur. Perhaps the single greatest strength of the social work perspective is recognition of parallel process. A supervisor who is confident and secure will not react defensively when issues arise. A supervisee will learn from this and not react defensively in her interactions with her clients.

Much has changed in health care in the past twenty years. However, the goals of helping professionals and paraprofessionals remain constant. People enter work with ill and disabled elders because they are motivated to help. The reality of "helping" is often disillusioning.

Gerontological Supervision
© 2008 by The Haworth Press, Taylor & Francis Group. All rights reserved.
doi:10.1300/5153_18

Old people are not always easy to work with. They are often ungrateful for help they wish they did not need. Yet there are enormous intrinsic rewards in a job well done. We hope that the social work perspective on gerontological supervision presented in this book will provide learning, insight, and growth to all levels of practitioners as they undertake this most important work.

Selected Bibliography

Atchley, R. "A Continuity Theory of Normal Aging." *The Gerontologist* 29, No. 2 (April 1989).

Austin, M. J. *Supervisory Management for the Human Services.* Englewood Cliffs, NJ: Prentice Hall, 1981.

Austin, M. J. and Hopkins, K. (Eds.). *Supervision As Collaboration in the Human Services.* Thousand Oaks, CA: Sage Publications, 2004.

Beaulieu, E. M. *A Guide for Nursing Home Social Workers.* New York: Springer Publications, 2002.

Bennett, R. and Gurland, B. (Eds.). *The Acting-Out Elderly: Issues for Helping Professionals.* Binghamton, NY: The Haworth Press, 1983.

Berengarten, S. "Identifying Learning Patterns of Individual Students: An Exploratory Study." *Social Service Review* 31, No. 4 (December 1975).

Berkman, B. and Harootyan, L. (Eds.). *Social Work and Health Care in an Aging Society.* New York: Springer Publications, 2003.

Binstock, R. and George, L. *Handbook of Aging and the Social Sciences.* 5th ed. San Diego, CA: Academic Press, Harcourt Brace Jovanovich, 2001.

Birren, J. and Schaie, K. *Handbook of the Psychology of Aging.* 5th ed. San Diego, CA: Academic Press, Harcourt Brace Jovanovich, 2001.

Brink, T. L. (Ed.). *Clinical Gerontology: A Guide to Assessment and Interventions.* Binghamton, NY: The Haworth Press, 1985.

Brody, E. M. *Long-Term Care of Older People: A Practical Guide.* New York: Human Sciences Press, 1977.

Brody, E. M. "Parent Care As a Normative Family Stress." Donald P. Kent Memorial Lecture presented at the 37th Annual Scientific Meeting of the Gerontological Society of America. San Antonio, Texas, 1984.

Bruce, E. and Austin, M. "Social Work Supervision: Assessing the Past and Mapping the Future." *The Clinical Supervisor* 19, No. 2 (2001).

Burack-Weiss, A. "Clinical Aspects of Case Management." *Generations* 12, No. 4 (Fall 1988).

Burack-Weiss, A. and Brennan, F. *Gerontological Social Work Supervision.* Binghamton, NY: The Haworth Press, 1991.

Busse, E. and Blazer, D. *Handbook of Geriatric Psychiatry.* New York: Van Nostrand Reinhold, 1980.

Butler, R. *Why Survive?: Being Old in America.* New York: Harper & Row, 1975.

Butler, R. and Lewis, M. *Aging and Mental Health.* St. Louis, MO: C. V. Mosby Co., 1983.

Gerontological Supervision

© 2008 by The Haworth Press, Taylor & Francis Group. All rights reserved.

doi:10.1300/5153_19

Cantor, M. H. *Social Care of the Elderly: The Effects of Ethnicity, Class, and Culture.* New York: Springer Publishers, 2000.

Caspi, J. and Reid, W. *Educational Supervision in Social Work: A Task-Centered Model for Field Instruction and Staff Development.* New York: Columbia University Press, 2002.

Cox, E., Kelcher, E., and Chapin, R. (Eds.). *Gerontological Social Work Practice: Issues, Challenges, and Potential. Binghamton, NY: The Haworth Press, 2002.*

Cummings, S. and Galambos, C. (Eds.). *Diversity and Aging in the Social Environment.* Binghamton, NY: The Haworth Press, 2004.

Edelson, J. S. and Lyons, W. H. *Institutional Care of the Mentally Impaired Elderly.* New York: Van Nostrand Reinhold Co., 1985.

Germain, C. and Gitterman, A. *The Life Model of Social Work Practice.* New York: Columbia University Press, 1980.

Getzel, G. "Social Work with Family Caregivers to the Aged." *Social Casework* 62, No. 4 (1981).

Getzel, G. and Mellor, M. J. (Eds.). *Gerontological Social Work Practice in Long-Term Care.* Binghamton, NY: The Haworth Press, 1983.

Gitterman, A. and Gitterman, N. "Social Work Student Evaluation: Format and Content." *Council on Social Work Education* (Fall 1979).

Gitterman, A. and Miller, I. "Supervisors As Educators." *Supervision, Consultation, and Staff Training in the Helping Professions.* Ed. F. Kaslow. San Francisco: Jossey-Bass, 1977.

Goldstein, R. "Institutionalizing a Spouse: Who is the Client?" *Journal of Geriatric Psychiatry* 16, No. 1 (1983).

Greene, R. R. *Social Work with the Aged and Their Families.* New York: Aldine·de Gruyter, 1986.

———. (Ed.). *Human Behavior and Social Work Practice.* New York: Aldine de Gruyter, 1999.

———. *Resiliency Theory: An Integrated Framework for Practice, Research, and Policy.* Washington, DC: NASW Press, 2002.

Hawthorne, L. "Games Supervisors Play." *Social Work* 20, No. 3 (May 1975).

Holloway, E. *Clinical Supervision: A Systems Approach.* Thousand Oaks, CA: Sage Publications, 1995.

Holloway, S. and Brager, G. *Supervising in the Human Services: The Politics of Practice.* New York: The Free Press, 1989.

Hooyman, N. R. and Kiyak, H. A. *Social Gerontology: A Multidisciplinary Perspective.* Boston, MA: Allyn & Bacon, 2004.

Horowitz, A. "Family Caregiving to the Frail Elderly." *Annual Review of Gerontology and Geriatrics.* Ed. M. P. Lawton and G. Maddox. New York: Springer Publishing Co., 1985.

Johnson, J., Sakaris, J., Tripp, D., Vroman, K., and Wood, S. "Role of Social Work in Adult Day Services." *Journal of Social Work in Long-Term Care* 3, No. 1 (2004).

Johnson, T. F. *Elder Mistreatment: Deciding Who Is at Risk.* Westport, CT: Greenwood Press, 1991.

Kadushin, A. "Games People Play in Supervision." *Social Work* 13, No. 3 (March 1968).

————. *Supervision in Social Work.* New York: Columbia University Press, 2002.

Kadushin, A. and Harkness, D. *Consultation in Social Work.* New York: Columbia University Press, 1977.

Kaiser, T. L. *Supervisory Relationships: Exploring the Human Element.* Pacific Grove, CA: Brooks/Cole Publishing Company, 1996.

Kane, R. and Kane, R. "Alternatives to Institutional Care of the Elderly: Beyond the Dichotomy." *Gerontologist* 20, No. 3 (1980).

————. *Assessing the Elderly: A Practical Guide to Measurement.* Lexington, MA: Heath & Co., 1983.

Kennedy, G. J. *Geriatric Mental Health Care.* New York: Guilford Publications, 2000.

Koeske, G. F. and Koeske, R. D. "Workload and Burnout: Can Social Support and Perceived Accomplishment Help?" *Social Work* 34, No. 3 (1989).

Kolb, P. *Caring for Our Elders.* New York: Columbia University Press, 2003.

Linzer, N. "Ethical Dilemma in Elder Abuse." *Journal of Gerontological Social Work* 43, No. 2-3 (2004).

Mace, N. and Robins, P. *The 36-Hour Day.* Baltimore: Johns Hopkins University Press, 1981.

Matorin, S. "Dimensions of Student Supervision: A Point of View." *Social Casework* (February 1979).

McInnis-Dittrich, K. *Social Work with Elders: A Biopsychosocial Approach to Assessment and Intervention.* Boston, MA: Allyn & Bacon, 2004.

Mellor, J. and Ivry, J. *Advancing Gerontological Social Work Education.* Binghamton, NY: The Haworth Press, 2003.

Miller, I. and Solomon, R. "The Development of Group Services for the Elderly." *Social Work Practice: People and Environments.* Ed. C. B. Germain. New York: Columbia University Press, 1979.

Monk, A. (Ed.). *The Age of Aging.* Buffalo, NY: Prometheus Books, 1979.

————. "Social Work with the Aged: Principles of Practice." *Social Work* 26, No. 1 (1981).

————. *Handbook of Gerontological Services.* 2nd ed. New York: Columbia University Press, 1990.

Moody, H. R. *Aging: Concepts and Controversies.* Thousand Oaks, CA: Sage Publications, 2002.

Munson, C. E. *Social Work Supervision: Classic Statements, Critical Issues.* New York: The Free Press, 1979.

————. "Style and Structure in Supervision." *Journal of Education for Social Work* 7, No. 1 (Winter 1981).

————. *An Introduction to Clinical Social Work Supervision.* Binghamton, NY: The Haworth Press, 1983.

Naleepa, M. J. and Reid, W. J. *Gerontological Social Work: A Task-Centered Approach.* New York: Columbia University Press, 2003.

Nathanson, I. and Tirrito, T. *Gerontological Social Work: Theory into Practice.* New York: Springer Publishing Company, 1998.

National Association of Social Workers (NASW). *Standards for Social Work Case Management.* Washington, DC: NASW Press, June 1992.

National Association of Social Workers (NASW). *Code of Ethics.* Washington, DC: NASW Press, 1999.

Palmore, E. *Social Patterns in Normal Aging.* Durham, NC: Duke University Press, 1981.

Parsons, R. J., Hernandez, S. H., and Jorgensen, J. D. "Integrated Practice: A Framework for Problem Solving." *Social Work* 33, No. 5 (1988).

Perlman, H. H. ". . . And Gladly Teach." *Journal of Education for Social Work* 3, No. 1 (Spring 1967).

Quinn, J. *Successful Case Management in Long-Term Care.* New York: Springer Publishing Company, 1993.

Radol-Raiff, N. and Shore, B. *Advanced Case Management.* Thousand Oaks, CA: Sage Publications, 1993.

Rehr, H. and Caroff, P. *A New Model in Academic Practice Partnership: Multi-Instructor and Institutional Collaboration in Social Work.* Lexington, MA: Ginn Press, 1986.

Reynolds, B. C. *Learning and Teaching in the Practice of Social Work.* New York: Russell & Russell, NASW Classics Series, 1985.

Richardson, V. and Barusch, A. *Gerontological Practice for the Twenty-First Century.* New York: Columbia University Press, 2005.

Rosengarten, L. *Social Work in Geriatric Home Care.* Binghamton, NY: The Haworth Press, 2000.

Sadavoy, J. and Leszcz, M. (Eds.). *Treating the Elderly with Psychotherapy: The Scope for Change in Later Life.* Madison, CT: International Universities Press, 1987.

Shulman, L. *Skills of Supervision and Staff Management.* Itasca, IL: F. E. Peacock Publishers, 1982.

———. *Interactional Supervision.* Washington, DC: NASW Press, 1993.

———. "Supervision and Consultation." *Encyclopedia of Social Work.* 19th ed. Ed. R. Edwards. Washington, DC: NASW Press, 1995.

Silverstone, B. and Burack-Weiss, A. "The Social Work Function in Nursing Homes and Home Care." *Journal of Gerontological Social Work* 5 (Fall/Winter 1982).

———. *Social Work Practice with the Frail Elderly and Their Families: The Auxiliary Function Model.* Springfield, IL: C. Thomas, 1983.

Solomon, R. "Role of the Social Worker in Long-Term Care." *Journal of Gerontological Social Work* 43 No. 2-3 (2004).

Towle, C. *The Learner in Education for the Professions.* Chicago: University of Chicago Press, 1954.

Tsui, M. *Social Work Supervision Context and Concepts.* Thousand Oaks, CA: Sage Publications, 2004.

Vourlekis, B. and Greene, R. *Social Work Case Management.* Hawthorne, NY: Aldine de Gruyter, 1992.

Wagner, L. "New Strategies for Enhancing Employee Growth." *Provider.* pp. 22-33 (2005).

Walker, R. and Clark, J. "Heading Off Boundary Problems: Clinical Supervision as Risk Management." *Psychiatric Services* 50, No. 11 (1999).

Wasik, B. H. and Bryant, D. M. *Home Visiting—Procedures for Helping Families.* 2nd ed. Thousand Oaks, CA: Sage Publications, 2000.

Webb, N. B. "From Social Work Practice to Teaching the Practice of Social Work." *Journal of Education for Social Work* 20, No. 3 (Fall 1984).

Weiner, M. B., Brod, A. J., and Snadorsky, A. M. *Working with the Aged—Practical Approaches in the Institution and Community.* 2nd ed. Hormick, CT: Appleton-Century-Crafts, 1987.

Wilson, S. *Field Instruction Techniques for Supervisors.* New York: The Free Press, 1981.

Zarit, S. *Aging and Mental Disorders.* New York: The Free Press, 1983.

Index

Gerontological Supervision
© 2008 by The Haworth Press, Taylor & Francis Group. All rights reserved.
doi:10.1300/5153_20